BLOOM
Holistic Healing Methods For Sexual Abuse

♥ ♥ ♥

By Lyra Adams

© Lyra Adams 2020
All rights reserved.

Book reviewers, booksellers and librarians may quote brief passages and post cover image in a printed, online or broadcast review of book without permission from the publisher. Otherwise, no part of this publication may be reproduced physically or digitally, stored in a retrieval system, or transmitted in any form or by any means (including electronic, mechanical, photocopying, recording or otherwise) without prior written permission from the publisher.

Media info available at lyraadams.com

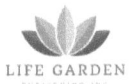

Published by
Life Garden Publishing Inc.
P.O. Box 333
Borden, IN 47106 USA

Table of Contents

About The Author 6

Acknowledgements 8

Introduction..10

For Friends & Family of Those Affected 12

1 - You Can Still Bloom 16

2 - What Is Sexual Abuse?...22

3 - Breaking Free..28

4 - Stages of Healing 34

5 - Your Voice 68

6 - On Auto-Pilot..78

7 - Feeling Comfortable In Your Skin............................86

8 - Taming The Dragon 96

9 – Addictions 106

10 - Recognize Your Transgressor 124

11 – Preferences 150

12 – Reconnecting 162

13 – Trust 194

PART II – Transforming With Nature 202

14 – Energy 204

    Chakra Energy Centers 207

    15 – Nature 222

16 - Subtle Power of Flower Essences 226

17 - Gems From The Earth 232

18 – Sound 242

19 - Mental Focus 250

20 - Self Forgiveness 260

21 - Self Love 266

22 - Changing Our World 268

Appendix 269

References 272

Images 274

About The Author

Some say she is a dreamer ... and that is true. Lyra is a dreaming empath, but so much more. She is an advocate and champion for those that have been victimized. She is a mentor to those who want to level up on their spiritual path. Lyra is affectionately known as the Queen of Synchronicity because she often experiences events way beyond coincidence. She states her "life is an extraordinary mixture of extreme blessings, divine intervention, and tragedies that often turn to triumph."

To date, her writings have focused on self-help within the holistic healing spectrum. She has been working steadily on a fictional series as well.

Lyra hosts the Podcast, *Breaking Free ~ Healing the Emotional Effects of Sexual Abuse* available on all major platforms worldwide. She is an advocate for males and females who are victims, survivors and eventually SUR-THRIVERS!

Lyra began calculating natal astrology charts for friends by hand during her early twenties. She was a participant in 1982-1983 of the meditation group made up of some of the same individuals as the channeled *Law of One* philosophy. Areas of lifelong interest are astrology, divination, channeling, meditation, herbs, flower essences, psychology and holistic healing. Lyra views many of these topics as tools for tapping into her favorite subject of all ~ consciousness.

Acknowledgements

So much of what comes to me is divinely inspired. My focus on the concept of blooming and the lotus flower rolled right out in front of me, bit by bit, as I took a stroll or even a nap. I am forever grateful to the Great Creator God for inspired guidance in this endeavor.

I also want to acknowledge my review team who gave me honest feedback and helpful suggestions along the way. They were a small team, but mighty!

Special thanks to Angela Warren whose impressions and suggestions allowed me to gauge reaction to the information contained in the text. Angela, you are a delight!

Special thanks to Nigel who has been with me from my first book and is a continued source of information and inspiration. If I ever make it across the pond, we will have to meet for tea my friend.

Special thank you to Geraldine Heil who shyly, but effectively, probed the work with the right questions and suggestions. Again, when I make it to Camelot land, you are one I would love to meet in person. You have been with me since the beginning!

Thank you to my home girls, Holly and Danielle. Holly, you served to give valuable impressions of the focus of the book and are always encouraging. Danielle, you are my little Aries fire girl, lighting my arse when I need it and a pillar of support for my work. I love you both!

Finally, thank you to my readers, followers and listeners of the *Breaking Free* podcast for giving me the opportunity to be part of your lives. I work for you!

Introduction

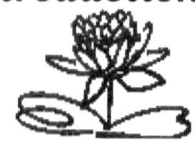

All persons affected by any type of abuse have opportunities through varied modalities to heal. Victims of sexual abuse often have experienced other abuses as well. These would include verbal, emotional and physical abuse. One of the main methods for assisting these survivors in making sense of what happened and how it could be carrying over into their present day life is cognitive therapy. This therapy is critically important as it allows each individual to come to logical conclusions about things. The emotional wounds held by trauma survivors are not always adequately addressed with this left brain approach. This writing focuses on the whole being or holistic approach to healing those emotional aspects held deep by those who have endured abuse. As a sexual abuse survivor, I have found these various methods of utilizing non-traditional healing modalities to be equal in importance to cognitive behavior therapy.

Many of the holistic methods listed in this book come directly from the earth. Nature, herself, can be an incredibly powerful healer when it comes to our moods and deeper emotions. Imagine now standing barefoot at the ocean's edge, sand between your toes, hearing the ebb and flow of the waves. Picture the blue sky, along with the sound of seagulls. Instantly, relaxation can overcome you.

Take a deep breath and transport your imagination to a lush green forest with tall pines. Smell the scent of the pine needles mixed with soil on the path you are walking. Reach out and touch the jagged bark of a tree. Place your back to the tree and take another deep breath. Allow the tree to help ground you emotionally. This is the power of nature.

At times, we can encapsulate bits of nature that are transformative carriers. Flower essences are one such substance that will be covered in many sections of this text. Another potential carrier of transformation is gemstones and crystals which will also be recommended for their potential healing properties.

Holistic modalities would not be complete without visiting ancient methods for connecting to our inner selves such as meditation and techniques for mindfulness. Technology is assisting us also in opening our vision of healing with methods.

Overall, my mission has been and is to introduce ways that can be utilized to speed healing and recovery from abuse trauma. Will one technique work and fix everything? No, it will not. It is likely the survivor will need to explore many methods of holistic healing and utilize those tools along with cognitive behavior therapy that is compassion based. Just as you require varied nutrients to live a healthy life, your healing may require many different components for you to achieve a state of not just surviving, but actually thriving in life. While those terms have almost become cliché now, they are currently the best description of the final goal for trauma victims. If I, as the author, were to invent another destination goal it would be wholeness — meaning that on a mental, physical, emotional and spiritual level, you are now restored.

This restoration is to your original potential when you were born into this life before cruel and predatory individuals came into contact with you. In this state, I certainly see you smiling — shining almost. This state moves you from powerless to powerful in navigating life joyfully on your terms. That is what I wish and visualize for you.

With much respect and love,
Lyra

For Friends & Family of Those Affected

For those of you that have never been sexually abused, the following thoughts and information are for you. Unfortunately, percentages for the number of males and females abused as children and adults have risen sharply over the years. I know it is very possible you do not want to live in a world where people are hurting others like this. There are many instances of sexual abuse, along with an epidemic level of human trafficking. This has evolved into separate components that sometimes overlap. There are people trafficked just for their internal organs – even children. There are people who are made into actual slaves in cages. There are people sold for sexual acts. People – human beings – have been turned into commodities like oil, sugar, illegal weaponry or drugs. If you think about it, this has been going on for hundreds, if not thousands of years. The methods and means by which it happens are the only things that change.

The traffickers and traders are people without normal empathy. They are trading humans as if they are crude oil, soybeans, sugar or coffee beans. The difference is this is a black market industry and it competes with illegal drugs. Often, the two are running side by side as drugs and human slaves are brought into a country or area together. Commodities are driven by supply and demand. It only works if there is a market for the substance. Many of the substances traded are addictive. Think about sugar – it is highly addictive. Having crude oil to fuel our lifestyles is equally addictive. It is addictions that also drive the black markets of humans and drugs.

I mention all of this because some have no idea the massive scale this is happening within worldwide. From the petty pimp on the street or in the strip club to larger organizations that traffic women, boys and girls ... there is a huge problem in our world that is underreported for a reason. It may interfere with the addictions of people who want the supply to continue. And that supply represents huge amounts of underground, untaxed money worldwide. This money equates to billions and billions of currency.

Many of these victims in bondage are confused. They may not even see themselves as victims. Sexual abuse does quite a mind job on people. They are changed on a mental level to believe this is their life and natural. Even if set free, they may continue on that path because this is what they believe is the normal thing to do. For those who have never been affected, it can really be difficult to comprehend someone having this stance. Yet, it is very real. Many human slavery victims are unable to break free from their environment. Many have been involuntarily drugged at times. Many become drug users to numb the mental, physical and spiritual torture they are under.

The focus of this book is on holistic methods of healing those affected by sexual abuse. However, we should all be aware that there are humans who are forced into other labor practices that have nothing to do with sex. These can include being forced or coerced to work with hazardous materials at the raw stage or exposure to same from the assembly of products from those substances. It can include low to no pay wages paid to individuals throughout the world. It can include unusually hard manual labor for long hours and/or child labor. All of this is a part of human slavery.

We must ask ourselves as consumers — are the needs for these products greater than the human rights violated to obtain them? To be more informed, watch the videos provided by the Blue Campaign of the U.S. Department of Homeland Security. I also recommended that you view this short list of myths about human trafficking at: https://www.dhs.gov/blue-campaign/myths-and-misconceptions

What can you do? First, make sure to stand against all forms of sexual slavery. This would include small children, teens and even adults who are being used in any way sexually against their will. Pornography is often a part of this. Support organizations involved with law enforcement that are directly targeting individuals involved in human trafficking and slavery. Support politicians who are actually working to bring these criminals to justice. Make sure they are not just talking, but actually doing what needs to be done to help more victims and bring perpetrators to justice.

Report possible abuse — it is often hiding in plain sight. Know what to look for. Just as airline employees have now been trained to watch for child trafficking, you can as well. Keep an eye out for small, unusual things as you travel or go about your normal endeavors. Human trafficking is occurring everywhere. It is very prevalent in the United States. Contrary to belief, it occurs in suburban and rural areas too — not just metropolitan areas.

The United States Department of Homeland Security has instituted the Blue Campaign which is designed to educate the public, law enforcement and others in recognizing signs of human slavery. You can download a printable card with potential indicators at their site: https://www.dhs.gov/blue-campaign/indicators-human-trafficking. Additionally, you may call 1-866-347-2423 in the United States to report suspected human trafficking. Victims may reach out for help by texting HELP or INFO to 233733 (BEFREE) — or they may call 1-888-373-7888.

Finally, if someone ever tells you they are experiencing sexual abuse, believe them and listen. Assist them in getting help from authorities and professionals. If someone tells you about their abuse that happened years ago, believe them and listen. Do not try to minimize it by stating that it happened a long time ago or is over now. For them, the effects have probably not ended. It took a ton of courage for them to speak of what happened. Just listen, be a friend. Let them know you will be there if they need someone to listen. You do not need to have the answers for them. Just be supportive and compassionate.

Finally, thank you for caring. On a hidden level, this horrific problem is affecting us all. Let's light this problem on fire and extinguish it for good. Together, we can stand for human freedom and sovereignty!

1 - You Can Still Bloom

Each of us is born with a capacity toward our own brand of greatness. Often, these attributes take time to appear in our lives. Not many of us are like Wolfgang Mozart, able to create pieces of music at four or five years of age. His sister, Nanneri, was also a child music prodigy. They traveled together as children throughout Europe entertaining the upper classes. Many find their true calling late in life after disastrous mishaps. Some choose to travel a safer road and live a simple life not exploring their true passions until later years. And then there are those that have been affected by traumatic events. These events required a time period of processing and healing before they could uncover their true selves and find inner fulfillment.

Infamous late bloomers include Ray Croc who founded McDonald's restaurants in his fifties. Let's not forget Harlan David Sanders (Colonel Sanders) who founded Kentucky Fried Chicken at the age of sixty-five. Anna Mary Robertson Moses (Grandma Moses) is a celebrated artist in fine and folk arts. She never began painting until she was in her seventies. Renowned chef, Julia Child, is another late bloomer. A. C. Bhaktivedanta Swami Prabhupada, the founder of the Hare Krishna movement did so at age sixty-nine.

Imagine being the parents of Albert Einstein. He did not communicate and speak until after the age of four. He was a high school dropout and could barely make it into a technical college. He worked much of his life as a clerk at the Swiss patent office, unable to obtain other employment after college. Yet, this man was a genius who later gave us many critical pieces of the physics puzzle regarding space and time.

It is my personal belief that each of us contains sparks of the divine to offer others whether it is within your own family setting, locally or globally. It may take time for it to fully bloom, but it always has the potential if nurtured. And, you deserve to be nurtured.

It would be very presumptuous to believe that any of these individuals had not experienced some sort of trauma or severe challenges in life. Perhaps, it was not sexual abuse, but maybe for some it was. Sexual abuse is a topic that many people hold inside and do not reveal. Sadly, there are so many events in life that can be traumatic to the human psyche. Hardly anyone escapes some form of trauma.

It is unknown where the spark of your consciousness began as it has most likely existed for eons. For simplicity, let's say you began as a seed with a hard outer coating that broke open and combined with other elements to form you. The very fingerprints on your hands are unique. No other human has your exact pattern. How can it be you live in a universe that is so vast with numerous things, yet everything has distinct differences? Snowflakes fall and look relatively the same. Under a microscope we see one frozen snowflake compared to another and their structures are quite different.

As much as you were born from your human mother, you also emerged from mother earth after being spread by the winds of father sky. Like some flowers, you have been stepped upon during your growth -- trampled in a thoughtless, greedy way. Yet, fortune is in your favor as you made it and survived. Sadly, those less fortunate had their petals, roots and stems completely destroyed.

When you hear that you are fortunate, it is easy for doubts to arise. You may be feeling stuck in the ground and unable to push yourself past the mud. Perhaps, you are afraid of what others will think, say or how they will treat you if they know your past. You were trampled, but you do not want anyone feeling sorry for you. You want them to think you are okay. Deep down, you know something is not right.

Pushed down in the muddy waters, you stay close to your roots. Things feel safe here. Everything above is unknown. Sometimes you feel that something bad could happen if you actually explore your real thoughts, memories and feelings. It is not so much other people you are afraid of … although sometimes that is definitely true. Could it be that you are most afraid of yourself?

At times, you smolder in the mud with anger for what cannot be fixed or expressed. The things that bother you are sometimes hidden from your sight. Often, you wonder what exactly has you so depressed. Something inside is not right and you know it. You feel you lack meaning and could be confused on what your actual purpose is. Often, there is a pervasive feeling of not measuring up to others or being good enough.

But look how resilient you are — how you have endured what many do not even want to think about or imagine. Listen to the wind. It is saying: You still have the capacity to bloom.

Enlightenment and rebirth are concepts that have been represented by the lotus flower for thousands of years. The lotus embodies how we grow and bloom. It also exemplifies breaking free from patterns on this evolving pathway to our better self. While many use the metaphor of peeling skin off an onion to shed parts that no longer serve us, the lotus flower is a truer representation of beautiful human beings touched by abuse and trauma in any form.

Trauma and abuse leads survivors into a dark place where things can be confusing. Personal identity is sometimes lost. Depression, unresolved rage and other heavy emotions weigh an abused person down, deep down in the boggy mud -- the same place you will find the lotus.

Beginning its journey as a seed soaking up moisture from the muddy waters around it, the lotus slowly forms roots and finally a tight bud. This bud stays tightly closed until it feels ready to reach above the water and unfold. Each set of petals open at their own time -- not all at once. As the lotus flower gradually pokes above the water, its beauty is revealed. The petals are usually pink or white in color and the center, when finally exposed, is always a yellow or light green. The petals are exquisitely clean and not affected by residue from the murky water in which they grew. This is due to two elements. First, the tightly wrapped bud prevents debris from entering while under water. Additionally, a waxy coating on each petal allows dirt to slide off each petal easily if it should come into contact. If we look at the center of the lotus as the soul of the flower and the petals as varying elements of its existence, there are many things to contemplate in relation to the human being and the lotus flower. The lotus also represents rising above negativity (or what we perceive as such) and overcoming adversity.

At times, people confuse the lotus with water lilies, both beautiful. Yet the lotus has some distinct attributes and is one of the most hardy flowers in the world. Its seed, which has a thick armor, can remain without water and bloom hundreds and in some cases thousands of years later. All that potential staying put for so long and finally, centuries later, its beauty is revealed. But at least part of the time, we find the lotus flower closed and withdrawn into the mud. And that is where we shall begin our blooming journey together -- staying put for a bit in the mud.

While you and the sacred lotus share enormous similarities, eventually, you realize that you and the lotus are one. When you become the lotus, you have taken on a brave journey to venture above the water. You have prepared yourself by developing your own set of armor that still allows your beauty to come through and allows the mud residue to slide off effortlessly. You have opened your petals and examined them carefully, looking for hidden patterns and things that no longer serve you.

In order to accomplish this, you must face the feelings you have been pushing down into the mud. These feelings have often been weighted down with sadness and it feels uncomfortable to allow them to bubble to the surface. Some of the feelings you buried are so red hot with passionate anger they could boil the mud around them. But you had to do this burying in order to cope with the day to day survival issues you found yourself surrounded by. There is a very keen part of you that knows these buried feelings are weighing you down and keeping you from the better life you want. It's called denial and all humans engage in it. It is almost an unspoken coping mechanism requirement of those that have been abused. If we did not engage in some denial, we would hit the world in such a raw way it would be difficult to navigate in any type of normal fashion. It would be like taking a walk in the cold arctic winds with no hat or head gear. We would be chapped, chaffed and perhaps frost bit.

Denial has been our one of our best friends buffering our experience for us. However, when we are ready to move out of an invisible misery that cloaks our life experience, we must unearth what our friend denial has kept buried from us. As we do so, we see that it can be messy dredging that muddy pond. It can also be tempting to push it all down again in an attempt to see no evil, feel no evil. Yet, I believe if you are hearing these words, you are ready to begin unfolding into the lotus that you are.

You are ready to let the sun shine on those parts of yourself that you felt could not be cured. No longer a victim, you are ready to drop the veil and seize the life that was partially stolen from you.

Denial was really good for a period of time. It allowed you to operate. When you first learned to ride a bike, you used training wheels. While this is not a perfect analogy, training wheels are like denial. It served you for a time. But after awhile, you are grown up and the other kids are looking at you and asking why in the world you are still using training wheels. If you ditched them and faced your fear, you could ride faster and farther. The training wheels are holding you back even though you feel safer on your bicycle by having them. But it does take a step of courage to get a wrench or screwdriver and remove those extra wheels you have relied upon. Once they are off, it takes more courage to get on the bike and ride, hoping you won't tip over without them. Dropping denial is the same way. It was necessary so you could get out on a bike initially. The extra reliance on it worked well for awhile. But now, you want to ride freely and that is going to require being brave and going through the motions necessary to do so.

As the lotus, you know that in order to fulfill your purpose and bring joy to yourself and others, you must still sometimes go deep into the darkness of the murky waters and look for new agendas or clues that could be stifling you in any manner. This healthy constant reexamination keeps you bright as you emerge again from the waters and drink in the rays of the sunlight. Before you, my friend, is every reason why you can rise from your past and spread your limbs toward the sun.

2 - What Is Sexual Abuse?

When I meet people or walk among others at an event or just along the sidewalk, I have a special knowledge that being a survivor allows me to hold. On a deep level, I realize each person has a story, one that many may never share with anyone else. Their stories may include health or learning challenges they have endured. It could encompass problems with their parents, brushes with the law, death of loved ones and it could also include sexual abuse.

What do we consider sexual abuse to be? In most countries, it covers a number of ways of acting inappropriately and often under force or violently. In some areas of the world, rape is condoned within certain classes or groups. A female who is raped in some countries may have the blame for the act put solely upon her. Even more unfair and hideous, she may be executed after such an event because she is now not a virgin.

Sadly, I receive messages periodically from victims that are in these types of situations in their country. Generally, there are no laws and no policing to keep these individuals safe. Their resources are very limited. Often, I am contacted by them through a Christian missionary project.

Sexual abuse comes in many forms. A broad definition would be that it is any type of intrusion into your mind and/or body that is sexual in nature. It can be subtle, yet significantly impact a person. It can be violent or very coercive. Sexual abuse can affect us in a myriad of ways and be the cause of much psychological distress.

Particular definitions would include, but are not limited to:

➤ Uninvited and inappropriate touch or fondling

- ➢ Coercive rape under duress
- ➢ Violent unexpected rape
- ➢ Sex trafficking
- ➢ Mind control or attempts at same
- ➢ Invasion of your privacy such as someone photographing, filming or recording you without your permission
- ➢ Someone sending you inappropriate things by mail, email, texts and messaging.

This book is for all genders. Sexual abuse is not a female only problem. This information is for all people who have experienced any type of sexual abuse.

Why Me?

Allow me to give you a brief synopsis of my story which I outlined in more detail in my first book, *Dreaming Synchronicity*. As a young teen with braces still on my teeth, I was raped repeatedly and sex trafficked. One of the lucky ones, the police found me and I was rescued. But I was covered in shame as I returned to my "normal life".

My family never spoke about the sexual abuse I endured. It was like it had not happened. In their minds, I just needed to go back to school and on with my life. They wanted me to fall into place, go to high school, college and be normal. But, I wasn't normal -- yet, I tried to be

I had deep issues that were stuffed down inside and they peeked out at times in ways that were not conducive to me. I couldn't live that normal life my parents wanted for me. I could not even live the life I wanted for me. I was directionless and sometimes unknowingly self-destructive.

When I was initially rescued, I did experience some inpatient care at a mental facility. This happened right after my horrible incident. While I was there, I do not remember pouring out my pain to anyone at the hospital. This was despite the fact that I had plenty of professionals working with me around the clock. I was just too ashamed. I was afraid to talk about what had happened in any detail. Plus, I did not trust anyone. Consequently, when I came home ninety days later from the hospital, I was not "over" what had happened to me. I was not healed at all.

Denial stayed with me from my teen years until my early thirties when I began to fight heavy depression coupled with an anger I would sometimes wake up with in the morning. I did not know who I was angry with. I was just pissed off. The subsequent depression made me very suicidal. Yet by this time, I was a single mom with two children and they needed their mother. I could not, would not do that to them. Suicide, no matter how depressed I was, could not be one of my options.

It was at one of my lowest moments that I sought professional help and I wish I had not waited so long. Those fifteen plus years I spent after being rescued from my pedophile pimp were rough and a little crazy. There were many wrong choices, promiscuity, and imbalanced living. Basically, I did not value me.

Without knowing it, I was a sitting duck and easy bait for sociopaths and those with other personality disorders. In a cloud of confusion, I was unable to see what was really going on with me. The funny thing is, I thought I was okay – until the depression and anger years later became out of hand. I moved about reacting to life instead of directing it. I believed my abuse was just something that had happened; happens to many; and I had "moved on".

But sludge was clogging the gears in my brain. As it picked up more debris along the way with my poor choices, there came a point when I could stand it no more. I had to break the negative, destructive patterns I saw myself engaged in. I wanted a good life for me and my children. I longed for a real romance with a partner who would love me – all of me good and bad. I wanted a partner who put me on a pedestal instead of the ones that started out well and eventually tore me down. I wanted financial rewards along with the freedom to be me. It took time, but I got all of it. It took work, but the rewards have been worth it. And, you know, I still have to work at it but not nearly as much or as hard.

I have experienced periods where I have slid back into behaviors I thought I was done with. Behaviors that threatened all the great things I had created and the uplifting way I had forged ahead in life. Why does this happen? You see, these feelings and experiences are grooved into our subconscious like an old record album. If we are not careful, the song will replay. Along the way, I found methods to help me. These precious tools are part of what I want to share with you.

In 2018, I wrote a memoir, *Dreaming Synchronicity: Journey of an Empath*. The book covers many things, not just sexual abuse. In fact, that is a small piece of it. More than anything, I attempted to show in the book how I shed patterns that were no longer serving me and how they developed to begin with. With my book published and available just about everywhere in the world, I thought I was done with this subject. In fact, I moved on to writing many other things. But, I got triggered! You know how that happens don't you?

My trigger was reading and hearing about the entire Jeffrey Epstein trafficking ring. To me, it seemed that the focus had been too much on the predator. In this case, I probably should make that plural since he had so many helpers and clients that also raped teens. I became agitated with the focus being on the predator. There was too much talk about his island; how much money he had; how he was slapped on the hand and put on work release in Palm Beach, Florida where he would go down to his mansion and work in his office each day still raping daily.

There was too much talk about his ranch in New Mexico and even his plans to impregnate women and make his own human race. Next, it was a debate about whether he was murdered or committed suicide. How about the possibility of neither? You never know in today's world.

All of this was too much for me because I wanted to know about his victims. I wanted to know how this impacted them. I wanted to find out where they are in their recovery. How it has changed who they were into who they are now. I want them to be able to speak if they choose to. Some want the victims to have their day in court and I understand that. Where possible, all victims should be able to have that partial closure. But it is only a stepping stone toward healing. It is those that were abused that need to be focused upon and helped. This is following them their entire lives; just like my experience follows me.

Now the victims do not have another outlet to right the wrongs they endured -- because he's flown the coop. Civil lawsuits for monetary awards could prove fruitful. Money helps but it does not fix the issues survivors struggle with. It could help in paying for psychological counseling, or moving to create a new life or identity. It could help with education costs. But the sticky residue that hangs on still must be addressed with or without money.

Most of us were not abused by someone so high profile, but some were. For me, my predator was just a lowly guy on the trafficker totem pole. Even though they arrested him, nothing happened to him legally. No, nothing happened and I spent all those years silent with my pain and shame shoved down so deep I didn't really know it was there or how it was affecting me. I guarantee you he just went back to finding more victims and doing his job as usual.

With this triggering event, I had to ask myself: Who is going to help these people that have been profiled, coerced, tricked, raped and violated? Who will help the child victims out there being trafficked each day and night in this world? Because, when their keeper is done with them, it is likely one of two things happens: they live and are given their freedom or they are killed.

In my book, *Dreaming Synchronicity*, I made a prediction toward the end. I stated that if there is one thing we could all come together on – one issue that should reach across all political and religious persuasions it is this: We must protect the children of this world. Truly, they are the future. I will add that we must also help those that have endured abuse heal because if they don't they will either self-destruct or hurt others. We need help from the entire rest of the decent population on this planet to stop these crimes against human beings.

All of this compelled me to do something – whatever I could – to assist others in healing. I have now spent many years on this healing path and I am grateful to travel this journey with you. By sharing the tools and knowledge I have accumulated and continue to mine for, we help heal the world as we heal ourselves. Nothing pleases me more than helping other survivors bloom!

3 - Breaking Free

I was listening to a music mix and *Crucify* by Tori Amos began playing. I purchased Tori's music as soon as it was released in the 1990's. Years later, I attended two of her concerts. To say that I resonated with it would be very accurate. In this particular track, Tori spoke of the price we pay when we hold onto a victim or martyr frame of mind. In the early 1990's, I was fully engaged in my healing of the past, yet had no real idea what I was doing or where the process was taking me. When I listened to the song at that time, I felt validated with lines like "nothing I do is good enough for you". As I listen to the words now, what stands out to me is breaking free from the tragic residue that can ensnare and trap us. In my mind, I see a human trapped by a thick, sticky substance glued to a brick wall. Their face is opaque with the glue trapping them. They cannot easily breathe. This victim needs to make just the tiniest tear in the glue to begin the process of breaking free.

I realized listening to the same song I resonated with thirty years ago, that I now finally understand things on a different level. I look back on all my experiences in a new light. I grew out of that victim stance. I also traveled through the survivor phase, but now, I find myself in the warrior mode. I cannot tolerate living what days I have left here, in this body on this planet, not doing something no matter how small it seems to help those that have been victimized and enslaved. Because I know even if they are lucky enough to break free from the tethers of their captors, they are then prisoners of their own minds. So, what difference can I make to bring solace, peace and even victory to these men, women and children? This is my quest.

In this chapter, we will discuss some of the telling signs of someone who has not healed from sexual abuse. Keep in mind there are those who have partially healed, but still have work ahead of them. You do not need to have the majority of these symptoms or behaviors — only a couple to qualify. The longer the abuse occurred and the younger the age it happened, usually lends to more symptoms or behaviors being present.

Hypersexuality and Promiscuity - for some sex abuse survivors, having a sexual encounter with a new person is almost like shaking hands. In their mind, they hold an unconscious belief they are somehow obligated to have sex with people and this is normal. Due to a lack of real intimacy, sex is really no big deal to them. But, think about all the risks. These survivors sometimes dress very provocatively or wear little clothing. There may have been a reward mechanism between the victim and their predators when they were undressed or dressed in a certain style or manner which makes them continue to follow this routine. For women, this may be the only way they feel pretty. For men, this may be the only way they feel attractive.

Even if the hypersexual survivor settles down with one partner for a time, it will be a rocky romance for a number of reasons. First, the relationship is likely based primarily on physical attraction and the sexual act. Since a more complete healing has not occurred for the survivor, they still operate mentally from a victim mode much of the time. Risky behavior, especially when without a partner, is prevalent. This could include many one night stands.

Hyposexual survivors may become celibate for long periods of time in their lives or permanently. Individuals reacting to their abuse in this manner will probably dress very conservatively and perhaps wear more attire than is needed. Their clothing may be that which is very standard without anything standing out in order not to call attention to them. They just prefer to fade into the wallpaper and not be seen. While this survivor does not encounter the risks that one with hypersexuality would, they are still not healed. Their choice they are making is an emotional response to trauma wounds that still need to be healed to live a very different, better life — whether that includes sexual relations or not.

If your sexual predator(s) were female or male, you may both hate that gender and strive to avoid them as an adult or you may gravitate toward receiving attention from that gender because you see that as being valued in some way.

Another sign there is healing to be accomplished is when the survivor is experiencing anger, depression or both. Many sexual abuse survivors internalize anger they feel at their predators toward themselves. This results in depression because they do not have a healthy way to express that anger. Unfortunately, some sex abuse survivors act out their anger on others in various ways including becoming abusers themselves. It is as if they abuse others, it will relieve the inner turmoil they feel. Ultimately, it does not.

Survivors with trauma wounds can be afraid at odd times for no real reason to justify it. These are usually emotional memories and triggers activating them. Survivors often suffer from Complex Post Traumatic Stress Disorder (C-PTSD). They can be easily triggered with familiar words, smells, sights or sounds that somehow relate to their trauma. Abuse memories are stored in a vault of our mind and are not always readily accessible to us. When certain things occur that mirror our trauma abuse, some of the contents of the vault can be released resulting in these emotional triggers.

Many survivors in need of healing and still experiencing victim mode need to be in control of their surroundings. This makes them feel safer even if it is an illusion. It also makes it difficult for them to form relationships. It is so understandable how they can feel this control is important to them, however.

Another symptom of work to do is lack of empathy for people who "cannot get it together" as well as you believe you have. After all, you've been through all this trauma and you go on working and living. Why can't they who have never endured such abuse?

Development of extreme boundaries where an individual is uncompromising or unbending is a signal of coming from victimhood. Conversely, having poor boundaries where others can walk all over them as they strive to find their value through pleasing others is the same problem — just a different end of the spectrum.

Victims may feel that "If people really knew me, they would not like me" — as if there is something sinister and wrong with them. Victims may denounce all religion and spirituality and declare an atheist stance. This is very common when one or more of their perpetrators came from a particular religion. In the alternative, they may become extremely devout with a particular religion, philosophy or spiritual practice. Victims can also be prone to joining up with others who are in what many would consider a cult.

Toxic relationships are very common where you cannot seem to break free from the other person. If you are in a codependent mode, you almost always attract friends or lovers that are suffering from narcissist personality disorder or other maladies such as anti-social (sociopaths) or worse, psychopaths.

Here are more signs of still operating from victim stance:
- Staying busy all the time to avoid looking at you in a real deep way.
- Trouble with the law.

- Ongoing issues with family dynamics that involve acceptance and trust.
- You begin having flashbacks which you quickly push away
- Panic attacks and anxiety
- Suicidal thoughts and/or attempts
- Addictions
- Feeling disoriented about sexual identity and/or preferences
- Body image issues
- Self mutilation
- Lack of self worth
- May find you gravitate to occupations such as exotic dancing, pornography, prostitution.

There are numerous advantages to letting go of the victim role through therapies of many sorts. Statistics show those who stay in this mindset often are raped or abused again. This can also be verbal and physical abuse. It is like you are sending out a signal and the predator can sniff you out. The best way to keep this from happening is by working on your healing with professionals and on your own as well. This healing journey will require you to take an active part for sure. When you leave victim mode, you will move into full survivor status. Once you feel fully empowered with your experiences and new knowledge, you are able to move into warrior mode where you will be the director of your life.

Notes To Self

4 - Stages of Healing

Do you remember the moment you knew you had to address what happened in your past? What stage of recovery do you believe you may be at now? Many are just coming out of the denial that plagues everyone who has endured sexual abuse. Yet, someday – something happens that makes us realize we are not over it. In fact, if we really look at ourselves, we realize this was never dealt with fully.

Your experience could be buried because you did not want to face it. Often, the family and friends who knew of it did not give you the right kind of support. This may not be their fault, but more of an inability. People often do not know what to do when someone they love has endured rape and other such crimes.

You may think to yourself: I am a survivor. I have gone on with life. It doesn't matter now, right? You <u>deserve</u> to let this matter. When you heal, your life will change in miraculous ways for the good. I and many others can attest to that. Start now ... where you are ... no matter how advanced or behind you feel in your recovery. Along the way, be gentle with yourself and have patience. Healing takes time. It takes wanting it too. Sometimes, we have to hit a certain plateau or a bottom that calls out for us to change our direction. So, if you're not ready, set this information aside on a shelf. Reach out and grab it when you are.

If you are experiencing problems with trusting others, this will be an area to work on during your healing journey. If you have difficulty communicating effectively with others, this is another aspect. If you have emotions fluctuating frequently and cannot seem to regulate them well, this is more healing that must be done.

There are various stages to healing and they can be different in length for each individual. One important step is allowing denial of the events to stop. If your life is not working, you have to look at what happened. The moment you do that, you have made a giant leap across the Grand Canyon of your recovery.

Many survivors want results that are very instantaneous. They can be under the impression that if they go through certain programs or spend three months in therapy that they are done and life is going to be different. In rare cases, this could be true. And who can blame anyone for wanting to get the work over quickly? In some cases, it could be things will be very different after three months of therapy and inner work. You should be seeing some results. Just realize you may need to keep going with your healing journey for awhile. Starting small can sometimes give better long term results.

If I try to rush through and read a large textbook on physiology or space science, there is no way I will take in everything. I will only get the general idea of it and I'm not going to be very good at the details of the subject matter. With my learning style, if I do not pause and look up definitions for the words I do not know, I may be wasting my time. Sure, I will pick up some facts and have a general overview of the subject matter, but I am really not mastering the material. The same goes for recovery. Your desire to speed through this is normal. Everyone wants to get out of pain and get to the reward. You have to consciously ask yourself to slow down and go through all the motions of healing to get to the prize.

The trauma that you are overcoming may have only happened in an instant but it left some residue that takes awhile to shed. If you imagine a rainbow with a pot of gold at the end, you have to begin at the bottom on one side and make your way up. As you climb, you build strength and momentum. Once you reach the top or pinnacle, you will find the rest is a faster downhill run to reach the pot of gold. Much of the fun is actually in the journey as you uncover the beautiful flower that you are and bloom.

There are external things that can help speed up recovery. These include help from therapists, medical personnel, if needed, and holistic approaches added for a further boost. Your therapies are like shots of Vitamin B along your path. They produce important healing moments and allow changes in your perception and thinking that is conducive to your ultimate happiness.

In this book, I use the analogy of blooming like the lotus. Sprinkled throughout this body of work are certain flower essences that can assist you on your healing path. Years ago, I befriended a lady who became a mentor and teacher to me for a period of time. Although she was much older than I, she seemed eternally youthful in a remarkable way. I loved so many things about her — her gentleness, magic and knowledge. She was especially proficient with flower essences, but adept at many other things as well. From this friendship, I developed a keen trust in alternative ways of healing. Learning that all disorders stem first from our emotional bodies and then pass to the physical has dampened my ability at times to be one who stays only with conventional ways. My personal feeling is that both methods, combined thoughtfully, are powerful.

I will tell you about specific flower essences which can help you heal and assist in correcting emotional states of mind. If you choose to explore these wonderful drops of nature, chapter 16 will give you a fairly thorough introduction. You will also see why flower essences are different than most tinctures and essential oils. The overall idea you should know about these essences is the three or more levels they work upon in humans. Flower essences are extremely beneficial as they work on the entire mind/body/spirit complex. The signature of each essence is so light as to feel almost invisible. However, the intensity of healing they can produce has been reported as profound for many people, me included. This is because flower essences work on a vibrational level that affects the whole being. We will speak more about energy vibration later.

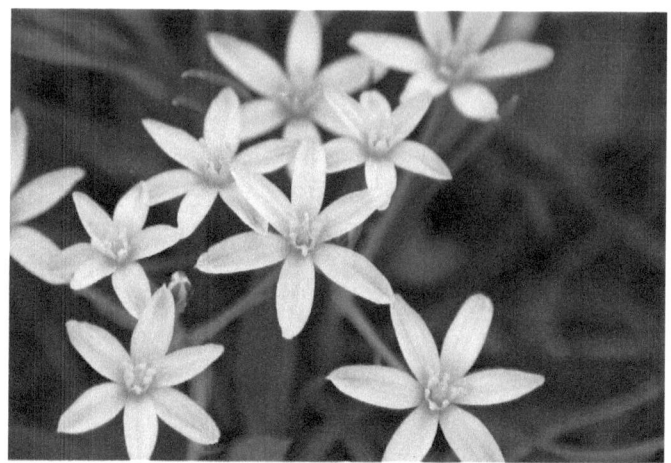

One of the best overall flower essences for people who have endured trauma is the Star of Bethlehem (Ornithogalum umbellatum). This flower has six petals which are all basically the same size resembling an actual six pointed star. It is beneficial for helping one to realign things that have become out of balance from traumatic events — especially recent happenings.

For a more thorough application of flower essence, it is not surprising that Lotus (Nelumbo nucifera) reigns supreme. Some flower essence practitioners view lotus as a magic elixir that helps to repair much for each individual. The very powerful lotus flower essence can be used for many remedies. Any aspect may be treated with this essence. Lotus can be used as a booster in another flower essence preparation as well. This flower essence gives relief to emotional challenges and brings the chakras into alignment. Lotus can help rid the body of toxic states that can block vibrational remedies from working effectively. When you cannot find this flower essence, Mango (Mangifera indica) works much like it. The flower essence of mango is not as potent and broad spectrum as lotus, however. It is interesting to note that fasting on mango juice or taking the flower essence for thirty days or more increases telepathic abilities. Mango opens you to the ethereal regions of your body. It also assists in repairing neurological tissue and slows aging. In its own right, mango flower essence is one of the most potent for spiritual growth.

Another flower essence for those that are facing challenging therapy is garlic. This is the essence of the flower so there is no garlic odor. Different flowers ranging from whites to purples bloom on garlic plants. One of the most notable things about the structure of those flowers is they remind me of an elegant reproduction of the brain.

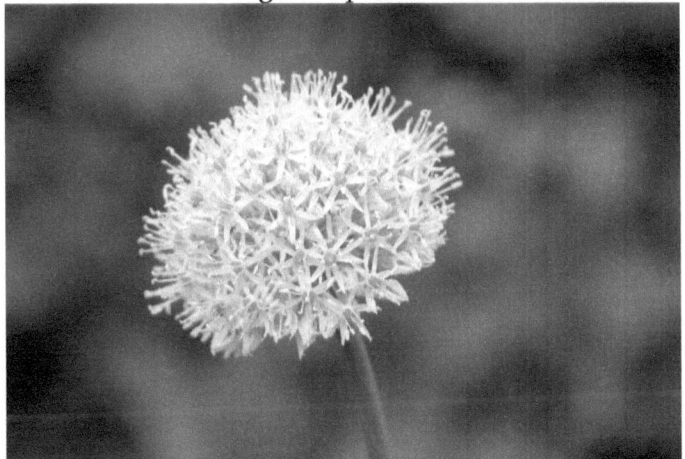

There are numerous flower essences, holistic therapies and gems from the earth that can assist you in each stage of your healing. Let us begin where we all do on this journey as we let down our guard and embrace our emotional wounds.

Denial

It can be difficult to choose which aspect of healing from sexual abuse to begin with. Where do we start in our journey toward healing trauma when there are so many facets to look at? Breaking it down, I thought back to my own experience of beginning the healing decades ago. I saw a picture of a young woman who, in many ways, had taught herself not to feel. Now, this does not mean I did not feel physical pain if I injured myself or emotional hurt from disappointments. Of course, I did. No, it was my reaction to events that I remember. Whenever something happened, I quickly attempted to mitigate it by silently declaring in my mind that I would get over it; would not let it hurt me. I was strong. I could handle it. After all, that is how I had handled my sexual abuse.

Instead of dealing directly with the cause of hurt or allowing myself to feel pain or emotions, I pushed them. In my mind, I was pushing them away from me. In reality, I was stuffing them deep inside. They fermented there, alongside all the other feelings I had placed deep inside me.

What did this look like on the outside? Close to the time I began recovery, a friend said to me rather bluntly, "you don't have normal compassion for others." I felt jabbed when she said this. In my mind, I thought I was a compassionate soul. I didn't argue, but instead made a point to really observe myself over the next few weeks. Was I hard on others? The answer was yes, at times I was.

By analyzing what my thoughts were in situations where people would or should normally feel compassion, I realized something about myself. Because of the abuse I had endured, I felt that others who were in a trying situation were just being cry babies. I truly had a "you better pull yourself up by your bootstraps and go on..." mentality. I lived that mentality each day. Not only was I hard on others, I extended that same attitude toward myself. I tricked myself into thinking that I met life with courage, yet I was a huge coward. I was afraid to deal with the things eating at me that I could not even see because they had been shoved so far in the dark.

This frame of mind was not serving me. As I trudged forward in life, I was making a lot of mistakes. Most of them were the same things or a variation of them over and over again. This happened with jobs, relationships and my general ways of living. The more I cut myself off from my true feelings and put on a false armor, the worse my life became, even though I was succeeding on some levels.

Denial is a natural mechanism built in to all humans to allow us to feel safer so that we can move forward with life. It is an excellent protection device for things we just cannot seem to handle at the time. When engaged in denial, we spend time saying things are not there, when they are. We refuse to acknowledge them because that may require something of us that is too much of a toll for where we currently are. During those times, we need that safety mechanism in place. It is no different than how our bodies go into physical shock. Shock is a protection that happens automatically to numb our senses. We don't tell our bodies to go into shock, anymore than we told ourselves to engage in denial. Our mind creates denial that naturally kicks in for us because it is painful to look at what happened.

The problem is that denial can become a way of life. Once you rely on it for coping with a traumatic event, you may find yourself engaging in it about many things. It becomes a way that is not true to us or others.

Denial reinforces the need for secrets. Secrets carried for years become such a burden they can make you ill. They can even make you want to harm yourself. In the medical field, denial like this is called experiential avoidance. Basically, it is the avoidance of thoughts, feelings, memories, physical sensations, and other internal experiences—even when doing so creates harm in the long-run. A study conducted in 2001 at Temple University by Marx and Sloan showed out of 99 survivors of child sexual abuse that experiential avoidance has a role in the development of psychological symptoms (Marx & Sloan, 2002).

Often, we are afraid if we open up and really think about something that we have been avoiding, it will make our life so different in a way that we fear. Change is difficult for many and it feels safer to remain in denial, sticking our head in the sand about things. And this happens to all humans. Yet, you are hearing these words and that means you are at least willing to take a peek. It means you know you may have something that needs fixing and healing. Denial is so pervasive in our society that we may not realize we do it. Here are some indications denial may be a friend you have that you don't know about:

> ➢ Frequently making excuses about the unacceptable behavior of others or ourselves.
> ➢ Not checking in with yourself about how you feel.
> ➢ Unable to be fully present in your feelings for a few minutes.
> ➢ Rationalizing that something is not that bad, when it really may be detrimental or unacceptable.
> ➢ Tolerating situations you do not need to tolerate
> ➢ Purposely staying away from others who may point out what you are avoiding. This includes not seeing people you have known for a long time that care about your best interests because you don't want to look at that right now. You may also fear they will have certain judgments about you.
> ➢ Trying to find blame in situations you are enmeshed such as when you have a push/pull situation or disagreement with someone. Are you in denial about something there? What do you need to see? Is the argument about something small and, if so, what is the bigger

issue behind all of it? What is the fear you feel behind all of it?
- ➢ Staying super busy so that you do not have to think about things you want to avoid.
- ➢ Taking up certain activities to the point of addiction to avoid something
- ➢ Any form of extreme risk taking or self harm
- ➢ Needing to end a work situation or relationship that is not serving the higher interests of each party. Instead of doing that, we remain in denial about the need for the split and spend our time trying to make it work.
- ➢ When someone shows you or tells you what you are in denial about, you feel angry with them. Instead, you kill the messenger not liking how they delivered the message to you, thereby bypassing the real issue that you are in denial about.

All of these ways of living are fear based. Secretly, you may fear that if you get out of denial and feel the pain that might be there, how will you handle that? I remember fearing that and even wondering if I might go crazy if I went through all those old memories I had stuffed down inside of me into the abyss of denial. Pushing away my feelings was denial, but the reality was that I hurt.

I did not want to feel emotional pain, so I developed a hard attitude with myself to avoid unpleasant feelings and carry on. Because I was not willing to analyze on a deeper level and deal with the things causing the hurt, I was stuck playing out the same scenarios in my life over and over again. Courage is required to leave denial and face things we have stuffed far away inside.

I found I was also battling particular types of family attitudes that had been passed onto me in a generational way. There was an unspoken rule in my family that was evident from everyone's behavior. That rule said: feelings are not that important. You need to think rationally about things. It took many years for me to realize that my feelings were the fuel for everything in my life and they were of critical importance.

As a survivor of any type of sexual abuse, you have at least been transgressed upon mentally. Most have also been transgressed physically. All have had a portion of their inner power stolen from them. All of this transgression leaves a type of void that feels too uncomfortable to bear. Denial that these unpleasant memories or traumatic feelings exist makes it much easier for you to move about in the world and carry on. Yet, at a certain point, it no longer serves you. In fact, it begins to hinder your progress toward your own best self.

Denial began as a friend protecting you from that which you could not handle. Yet, all those feelings you stuffed way down arise later to haunt and hurt you. While you may not know it is them calling your name, you find yourself feeling angry, depressed and out of sorts. But, you are not sure why. If you look at what you pushed away earlier and uncover just a bit of it, the healing process can begin.

Until you come out of denial that these past events are affecting your life, you will remain stuck. To move forward into a more beautiful life, you must do some work that begins with removing your barrier to admission. Your ticket to get inside the amusement park of life is letting go of denial — of being as truthful as you can at any given moment. And there will be times you can only drop enough denial to get your foot into the door. That's okay. With continued work and progress, soon you will have full admission to the park and perhaps even a fast pass. Admitting that you have issues from your experience is paramount to being the whole individual you deserve to be.

In our societies, there still remains a deep denial about the millions affected by sexual predators. Often, the emphasis is placed on the perpetrators who seem to never pay a very heavy price at all. The perpetrator dominates the news. The focus should be on gathering all energies to assist their victims. Could it be that as we move out of denial as a society where the abuse exists, we will facilitate healing and elimination of the crimes? Time will tell. I would like to see these perpetrators have to contribute significant monetary funds to pay for therapeutic treatments for survivors.

In this section, we have identified that denial can be a friend to us and that all humans engage in it at various times. We have seen that sometimes denial is the friend we held onto too long and keeps us from moving forward. The word *admission* has at its root "to admit". To change our life in a miraculous way, to gain admission into another reality where we are finally able to see more of the sun, we must *admit* that at the bottom of it all, we hurt. It can be scary to do this.

What does dropping denial and revealing our secrets mean for us? Will we have to experience those feelings? It is likely we will have to feel what we have put off. Will it be painful? Yes, it could be painful, yet cathartic and healing. And while you may do some of this by yourself, you absolutely need to be seeing a trained professional in conjunction with your healing. At the very least, you need someone who understands what you are going through and that you can trust with your life. Those people are few and far between and they may not know what you need at a particular time. That is why a trained counselor or even a sexual abuse survivors group would be very helpful.

For me, revealing my past to others began very small. Even though I had been seeing a therapist for the depression and anger I found myself experiencing, I never shared my sexual abuse with that counselor. The funny thing is I do not remember doing this deliberately. I truly was in denial that the events I went through were having any effect on me.

I later became so angry and depressed that I knew I was in a danger zone. It was at that point that I began seeing a psychiatrist. At some point during our therapy, it was there that I revealed my sexual abuse. I can say that it was painful, but I still wanted to tell myself that I was "past it" – that I had "moved on". Yet, revealing my secret was like letting a little bit of steam off the top of the pressure cooker. As time went on, more and more steam slowly escaped. It was a gradual progression of allowing things to surface.

You don't really know when the memories and feelings that were previously denied are going to pop up. It could happen while you are getting ready for work, eating dinner, watching a movie or taking a shower. Once you buy the ticket and say, okay, I'm willing to begin exploring and uncovering what I pushed down and away from me; that's when it will begin. It's like there is a little switch that goes off and it now tells that part of you it can begin to open the valve.

Generally, it will not happen all at once. However, I do remember when I began to come out of denial that I did have a couple of days where it seemed like a ton of memories were surfacing. I felt a lot of emotion and like I could not be around people on those particular days. I actually called in sick and took a mental health day for myself. I cried, read old cards and letters from that time period I had saved from my family, looked at childhood photographs and school reports. I grieved ….. for me.

It was difficult but it truly began to open me to new attitudes, opportunities and assist in transforming me into something greater than what I was before. It did not happen all at once. The shedding of denial takes time and the more gentle you can be with yourself while doing it, the better.

To continue to hide the horrible truth of what we experienced can cause physical illness over time, along with very challenging psychological issues. As it also affects us emotionally, we often make poor choices in life leading us down a path of self-destruction that is sometimes slow, sometimes fast. Our functioning in what we might consider normal social settings is also impaired.

When we begin to allow ourselves to open to the fact that the awful deeds committed against us truly hurt and were damaging, that allows us to be able to feel – yes feel. This is something we clam up on. We must ignore no more, but feel. While it may hurt at first, if we open up to another person in a safe space of speaking our truth, the burden will become lighter and lighter as time goes on.

I recommend that all survivors explore the depths of denial with a licensed professional trained in trauma work. Things that are not dealt with really can lead to depression and suicidal thoughts. So, it is really important to pick up the phone and make an appointment. You see, I am giving you guideposts along this journey, but I am not a licensed therapist. And, even if I were, I don't know your particular story. I just know that we have something in common. I am more like a friend who has traveled some of the same roads you have and can tell you what stops to make and which ones to pass up.

If you begin this journey or continue on it depending where you are in recovery, what can you expect? What is on the other side? From where I am now in recovery, I see that it allowed me to experience my feelings once more. This has helped me in so many ways. It has:

- Set me upon a healing path
- Allowed me to be forgiving and compassionate with myself and others

- Advanced me toward a wider, greater and strengthened connection with God
- Made me softer, not harder
- Made me truly care
- Made me more empathic
- Developed an inner fortitude and courage
- You are brave when you ask for help
- Made me a survivor or as some like to say, a SurThriver
- Allowed me to become unchained – to break free.

And that is what I want for you, friend. Keep going — you've got this!

Shame

When we share how sexual abuse affects people, we bring more awareness to those that have not been affected and could be very instrumental in assisting in changing the laws. We can never fully heal ourselves or this problem if we continue to push it into the dark. Sexual abuse cannot be taboo in our world conversation. For the individual affected, there is a level of embarrassment and shame to reveal their secrets even in a therapy setting.

It truly takes big components to heal:
- ❖ Courage – this is being strong or brave even though you are hurting
- ❖ Strength – staying true to your goals and path, even though you may falter at times
- ❖ Tenacity or Perseverance – a quality you call upon when it seems so difficult, but you do not give up
- ❖ Help From Others – you must be open to letting the right qualified people assist you.

It's hard to envision at times that you are capable of coming out of the shadows your shame has been hiding in. As someone who has traveled a very similar road, I understand you often have beliefs you are holding onto that support negative ideas about yourself. These can include core thoughts of not being good enough or that you can never fully trust people. Other thoughts could include:

- If people really knew me (or about me), they would not want to get involved.
- I am an emotional mess.
- I always eventually fail.
- Something always happens to mess things up.
- I will never find real love

Shame is the glue holding everything together in your physiological system. Without it, the whole premise that your life is playing out begins to fold like a house of cards or dominoes. Once you lift out the shame portion, you accelerate healing greatly. Now, it is one thing to just tell a person and this is very important to do, but it is another thing to still feel shame. That glue is heavy, sticky, old and hard. It needs to be literally pried out at this point depending upon how long it has been for you. Shame is always tied to secrets. It creates loneliness and isolation. You may still be around people but always feel like they do not really know the real you. They do not really know who you are and, if they did, you may not fit in with them anymore. So there is a fear factor of dropping our secrets. Most people would or do understand. They may not always know how to react. Many people may treat you different. They may treat you with kid gloves. Some cold souls may treat you with disdain. And if that is the case, you don't want those people around anyway because you have already been judging yourself for too long.

Shame is a judgment. It's an idea you came up with in your brain or that may have been put upon you by others. This false idea made you the one that did something wrong instead of your perpetrator(s). So, that is something to keep in mind always when we are dealing with shame. Shame needs to be dealt with and vanquished. You did nothing wrong when it comes to your sexual abuse. In life, everyone does things that are considered wrong. They make mistakes — something they could feel guilty over. Guilt is very different from shame, especially the kind of toxic shame that could be poisoning you.

As we let go of our secrets, as we speak about these subjects in an open way and with our children, we begin to eliminate much of the suffering that has gone on or could happen in the future. As long as we are uncomfortable and we keep treating the subject matter as secret, it is allowed to grow. People that would take advantage of others know this. When we let our secrets escape to the right people in the right circumstances, we heal ourselves. We begin the true journey of healing by allowing that to escape from us and sharing it somewhere else. Let's face it. What happened to you has been held secret. We all have secrets - things we choose not to share at all or only with some.

Shame is not always a bad thing. Healthy shame is temporary and correcting in nature. It is really more connected with guilt. Let's say your eleven year old niece lifts a tube of bubblegum lipstick from the store when you are with her. As you get into your vehicle to leave, you notice her with this item. You are certain she did not have it before. You question her and she admits to you that she stole it. You take her inside the store to return it or alternatively pay for it. You let her know how wrong this is and why. You let her know you will be telling her parents. It does not matter how much your niece pleads, cries or begs you not to tell, you let her know if you don't then you will be in the wrong for not being honest with her mother. She is going to feel healthy shame and/or guilt for doing something wrong. It will be important to not make your niece feel like she is a bad child or person, but rather made a very wrong decision.

There are many times when shame is misplaced – where we feel shame and have no real logical reason for doing so. This can especially happen around the subject of sex. We may think in the free, open societies we live in today that sex is no longer taboo. But certain aspects of it are still very uncomfortable for most. Depending upon what an individual has learned during their lifetime about their sexuality, shame can surround it for them. Often times, it is more like an uncomfortable embarrassment.

However, the shame that individuals who have been sexually abused suffer from is different. It affects their self worth. They feel less of who they really are as they carry this shame and it becomes like a poison inside. This is why it is often referred to as toxic shame.

Toxic, deep down shame plagues many, if not all, survivors of sexual abuse. For male survivors, the very core of who they are and their masculinity can be challenged on a deep level. Current statistics are that one in seven males will be sexually assaulted in some way. These figures only account for reported cases. We all know there are many cases unreported. Toxic shame can be combined with post traumatic stress and we may suffer fears of being abandoned; of not being good enough; of going crazy; losing relationships; or being a failure.

We may have a fear of emptiness; a fear displeasing others; a fear of being seen as a phony; a fear of not mattering; and a fear of being shamed by others. That is a whole lot of fears! Obviously, no one can thrive and be happy with fears weighing them down like this.

Shame is compounded if you were lured or tricked into the situation that led to your sexual abuse. This can happen in many different circumstances. It almost always involves extending trust to another who then violates that trust. If you are pressured into sexual situations in a workplace, it can be really difficult to speak up and speak out against this. There could be embarrassment and shame involved. Some people may not be your friend any longer. Some may be more of your friend than before admiring your courage to speak. Many children and teens are pressured in online social networking communities. Many times they are lured by an adult who has been grooming them for awhile, saying just the right things to earn their trust. Sometimes this adult is posing as a teen as well. Often with children, they are intimidated into not telling anyone. They carry their torture and shame a long time out of many different fears present.

Exploring what little we know at this time of Epstein's victims, they were scouted by other co-conspirators who profiled them first. They were looking for girls of a particular type for the pedophile ring. This included girls that had difficult home lives; perhaps not a lot of financial resources; and low self confidence. It was a bonus if the girls wanted to be models or movie stars. Just knowing this, can you see how these little girls cannot be blamed and should carry no shame for what they were eventually tricked into? I believe that shame can take on an even deeper level when you were coerced or tricked into sexual abuse. The reason is that many in society do not understand how people can fall under the spell of another like this. But psychopaths are skilled at these persuasive arts.

Perpetrators come in all different shapes, sizes, genders and ages. They can be almost anyone including:

- Other peers
- Parental figures
- Caregivers
- Teachers

- Religious leaders
- Scout leaders
- Camp counselors
- Relatives
- Strangers
- People who tricked us that we thought we could trust

Even a person that was stalked and physically attacked will question whether they could have prevented it. Perhaps they did not put up enough of a fight or a fight at all. Even an individual who was kidnapped will feel shame. All sexual abuse victims blame themselves to one degree or another. And the blame-shame cycle that ensues is a wheel we get on and seem to have a hard time getting off. Research shows that many types of violence experienced by people, not just sexual abuse, can produce shame and feelings of guilt (Aakvaag, et al., 2016).

It is time for us to stop being ashamed of crimes we did not commit. Shame that lies deeply within us often turns into self loathing and disgust. There is a part of us that feels worth much less than other individuals around us. Shame is what holds those feelings in place. What we end up doing is moving and operating in the world with those feelings showing up in strange ways without even realizing it.

For instance, you may not realize that you are not fully engaged when you speak to others or they speak to you. Your eyes may avert theirs. Your shoulders may be slightly slouched. Your walk, posture, even the tone of your voice gives out nuances to others that at a deep level, you do not feel good enough. Shame unknowingly cripples our self-confidence at times. Other people sense this.

In the alternative, we could feel compelled to push ourselves to extremes. We could have a false sense of bravado or ego trying to make sure others know our worth, even though we still do not really feel it inside and are hurting. Sooner or later, we have a mental split between the real core feelings and the exaggerated ego. When that happens, it could be called a crisis of sorts and the need for help from others is great.

Dr. Jerry Fishkin is a prominent neuropsychologist. He has spent decades treating persons for addiction and trauma. One of the things he noticed with his patients was that as they explored their background and hit upon any type of abuse or trauma, the patient either froze or bolted out of the office. They stopped coming and seeking treatment. From these reactions, he determined that shame is the cause of this behavior. He states that shame is something that lives in the basal ganglia of the brain. This area sits just above the limbic system in the brain where we have our seat of emotion.

People who have experienced trauma and abuse and have shame lying there, tend to have it grow over time. As it grows, it begins to try and control them through their internal self talk. Often, they never really feel good about themselves. I know I experienced this at a core level. During my years of recovery and even still, I will sometimes jokingly tell someone that I'm "just trying to keep my self talk good today". Self talk is the internal dialogue we have going on in our minds. It is the voice that says you are not capable, not good enough, cannot measure up, will never be on that level, etc.

I am grateful to Dr. Fishkin and his therapeutic approach to this. However, I really learned it for myself through spiritual practices such as affirmations. Guided visualizations helped me tremendously and this is because they work on that deep basal ganglia area. I did not know that at the time. I was just trying to feel better and get myself on a better road in life. When we imagine something with great emotion, it literally assists us in laying down new neural pathways to heal ourselves.

Dr. Fishkin also mentioned that there is often no pre-warning for shame attacks. He calls this toxic shame a type of "high jack of the system". He also says that we should not feel shame over traumas inflicted by others. Instead, those other people should feel shame. He says that when people have a shame attack, all they want is to escape or freeze in time/space (New Thinking Allowed, 2016).

We need to keep our self talk good and we can do that by listening to what it is saying at any given time or circumstance. Once we catch that negative little ninny saying the wrong things to us, we can correct it. Now, I often refer to the negative ninny also as your negative ego. It's a part of you that is almost like the little devil inside that wants to hold you back out of fear. The fact is, it comes from toxic shame.

Even those who have never been sexually abused can easily have this going on inside themselves. It could have occurred from bullying they were subjected to; wrong parenting methods; verbal abuse; physical abuse; anything that was traumatizing to their spirit. You came into this world as a beautiful whole being … and that part of you still exists. It is just being tamped down and held back with the same old recordings that are being replayed in your brain.

In conjunction with compassion based therapy, some of the suggestions Dr Fiskin recommended are:

- ❖ Writing a letter to your abuser or abusers. Remember, you do not have to send it to them. You can burn it, show it only to your therapist; do whatever you want with it.
- ❖ Journaling can be helpful for releasing feelings.

- Hypnosis can be another way to retrain the brain and lay down new emotions and thoughts.
- Getting angry and putting the blame back where it should be. You might hole up in a room and pound on pillows while you yell and cry in a safe space.
- Using guided imagery on your own or listening to positive visualizations through ear buds that assist you in raising your vibration.
- Using affirmations. One that helped me in the beginning was by Louise Hay and her story is very interesting as she was also a victim of sexual abuse.
- Gratitude journal – just writing down on a scrap piece of paper things you are thankful for.

Let's start with this: You are alive and you still have the chance to really thrive; you have comforts of some sort around you. You can easily make a list of things you take for granted that you can be totally thankful for. This retrains your brain to focus on the good. Over time, even a short amount of time, it brings results.

This is where we begin to heal the shame. If you are currently addicted to alcohol or drugs, you will need to work on detox before you begin healing issues around shame. You must detoxify your system first because the substances are affecting your brain.

For many reasons, it is easy to become addicted to substances. Do not be ashamed of that. But, do finally seek help. All of it is interrelated. If you do not have substance abuse you are dealing with and are ready to work on healing yourself through therapy, try to find a therapist that uses a compassionate approach or is using therapies for those affected by post traumatic stress.

We have to stop carrying the shame of the person or persons responsible for the wrongdoing. It is not ours – it belongs to them. If you are feeling their guilt and transferring it to yourself, try using the flower essences of eucalyptus or hyssop to alleviate this along with other therapies. With these two, hyssop is stronger for guilt and eucalyptus helps us to grieve for that which hurts us.

More than anything I want you to know that you must have lots of hope that things can and will change for you. What starts out slow as a tiny snowball can build as it runs downhill. Soon, you find your life changing in miraculous ways. It just takes you making the first steps, coming out of denial that these things are still affecting you, and releasing any shame you feel around the subject. Just letting go of those secrets can free you enormously.

What if this tragic trauma that was inflicted upon you builds you into a being that you never knew you could be? What if it encourages you to bloom more brilliant than you would have before? In some strange way, my quest to find a way to heal myself did that for me. That is why I ask you to hold hope for yourself and try. Try to go through the motions of healing even if you feel hesitant. Just take one step, then another, then another.

You are a human being that has tremendous value. You are here to do something and have a greater purpose. I cannot tell you what that purpose is but I know that your healing journey can reveal it to you. It may take time but the more you embrace the idea of healing your emotions and spirit, the faster you will see results in your life.

Please grab a notebook or journal and explore some or all of the following questions. This act will help you clear blockages to your healing. These are also in the Appendix for easy reference later.

- ❖ Are you hiding your true self in any way?

- Do you lie? Do you go along with others instead of expressing your real feelings because deep down you do not feel your ideas or opinion really count? Are you afraid to speak your mind? Do you lie to yourself?
- Do you have to cover up certain aspects of yourself or can you feel free to live more transparently for all to see?
- Do you fear rejection and does it keep you from having intimate relationships. Have you found yourself ending a relationship before it can get anywhere out of fear of being on the end of rejection later?
- Finish this sentence about your coworkers or friends: If they really knew me,
- Do you feel chronically lonely?
- Do you feel no one really knows you?
- Do you have a parent who shamed you? If so, do they still?
- Have you thought of harming yourself or suicide?
- Do you have self loathing?

Self Compassion

Sometimes we must ask: did I really put the responsibility where it lies? Do I spend time blaming myself for something I think inside such as should have known better or should not have done something? Are there people I can safely share my story with? Are there certain people I should never share with? How can I know who to talk to and who not to talk to? These are all important questions you must work through in your mind.

I recommend that you do not tell everyone about your past unless you want to and are very secure about doing so. It is more important during healing that you tell the right people. You need to know who those people are that would be best to confide in. You do not want others that will further question your story, like, "Oh, did that really happen?" "Was it really that bad?" Or, tell you a story that trumps yours — "Oh, that's nothing ... listen to this." You do not want to reveal your secrets to someone that tells you a lot of bad things have happened to people and you just need to move on. All of these responses show a lack of caring, empathy or even wanting to listen. It may be they feel overwhelmed with the information in some instances. They may feel as if you want them to do something about it, but they do not know what to do. Therefore, it is easy to say, "Look, shake it off. You have to get over this."

What they do not understand is that you have already been trying to do that in a number of different ways. Most of the time, you are denying yourself, blaming you instead of the perpetrator. By seeing this pattern you are engaging in with blame, you will release yourself from the unearned shame inflicted upon you. You have done nothing wrong! You did the best you could with where you were in the circumstance. So, have compassion for yourself. If others cannot provide that for you, at least know there are other survivors who certainly can understand where you are coming from. It is an unlikely band of brothers and sisters — one we wish did not exist. Yet, we must be here for each other with compassion and love.

Holistic Helpers

There is a gemstone used by some healers named Star Ruby. While this stone is used for different purposes to integrate higher energy frequencies into the body, it is extremely supportive for those inclined to self harm. A regular ruby gemstone has clear properties. Star Ruby is somewhat transparent but mostly opaque with six rays emanating from the center.

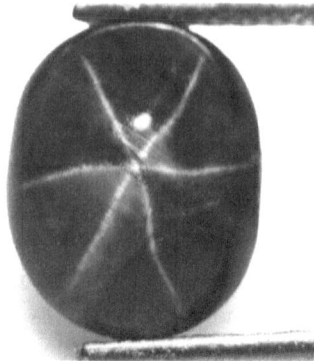

Rose Quartz is an excellent gemstone for promoting self love, something that is difficult for abuse survivors and necessary to build upon for healing. Keep it in as many areas as you wish!

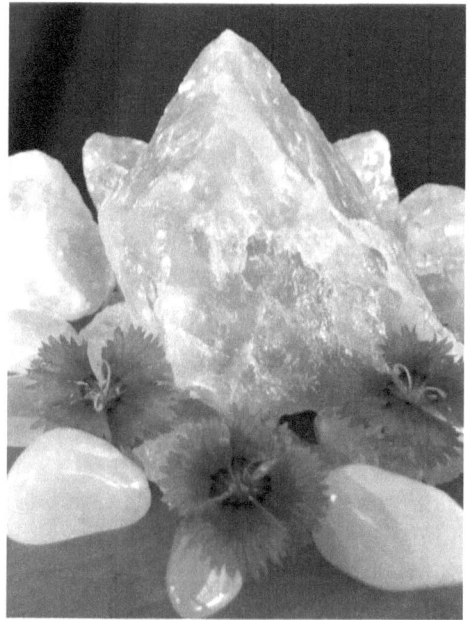

Reiki

This energy body healing method is powerful and has existed for centuries. The modern version, which is also just as potent, was revived by Mikao Usui of Japan. With this hands-on type of healing, Usui strived to re-create the healing methods of Jesus Christ. In later years, elements of Buddhism were intertwined with Reiki.

For over ten years, I have worked on my second degree in this discipline. That is because I have become distracted with other things during this time. I need to get back to it. It is like all skills, practice is required to not only keep your skill, but to become better at it. Once my teacher feels I am ready, I will study and be at the third master level of Reiki. At each training level, you must meet in person with your teacher and receive not only training, but attunements.

Another lady and I underwent attunement and training together for level one of Reiki. My first attunement was incredibly intense. I felt and saw light around me and I sat in pose with tears running down my cheeks continually. The emotion I felt was not sadness, but extreme joy — almost too much for my system to handle. Any ailments I had when I entered my teacher's home that day disappeared afterward including pain in my coccyx that I had been to my physician about. She had sent me for an x-ray at the hospital which showed nothing. All of our illness occurs on an emotional level first, then manifests into the physical. As I received this beautiful angelic like tuning, it dissolved many things for me on the emotional spectrum. It can be very helpful for healing trauma.

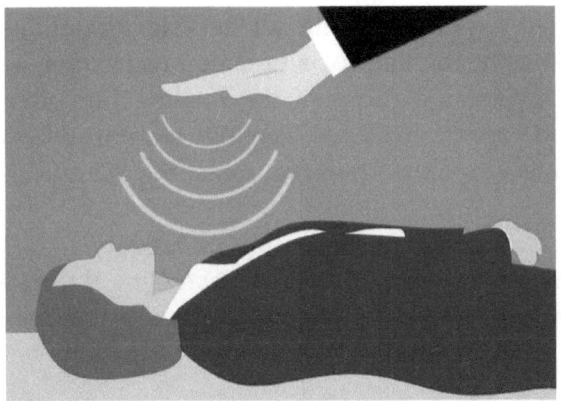

You do not need to become a Reiki practitioner, but you may want to go to one. Typically, you will lie on a massage table with your clothing on. Some Reiki practitioners may actually touch you lightly or lightly place their hand on certain parts of your body. I rarely do as I work with my eyes closed; feeling the energetic field of my subject which lies just inches above their physical body. By running my hands slowly up and down the entire body from head to toe in this energetic area, I come across certain areas that call out to me for love and attention. Those are the areas I focus upon. My volunteers often report heat in the areas I am healing, although I am not touching them. The healing power comes from God Source, in my opinion. The healer is simply a conduit to pass through, yet they must maintain a certain mind frame and tuning of their own energy complex to work effectively as a channel for the healing energy.

I have only seen my master teacher twice during the last decade to receive attunements, although I have run into her on a casual basis a few times. Being adept at this takes a serious look at long term becoming rather than fast results. Refer to the Recommended Reading section of the Appendix for more information on Reiki.

Other energy body work you may want to try includes acupuncture or acupressure if you have a fear of needles. My own experience with all healing modalities where I have sought the help of a holistic practitioner is that they and I determine more of the healing outcome than the method being utilized. Feeling comfortable with this person is very important and matching energies is a bonus.

Depression & Anxiety

One of the worst things about feeling depressed is that you lack the needed motivation or energy to make changes or do specific things that would ultimately help you to heal and feel better. Everyone who ever experiences the blues or depression knows this dilemma. It is a double edge sword! You know what might make you feel better, but you cannot seem to make yourself get there. You are just not at a place of being healed enough that you can. Other feelings and thoughts are weighing heavily upon you. You may be embroiled in situations that are more challenging right now. I understand. It is okay to be in that spot. We are all in a state of becoming and there is no judgment whatsoever.

Please realize that you might be in a pattern of beating up on yourself. While I would love to see you move away from doing anything like that, I realize that all of this is a process. Goals and working toward the future could seem either unimportant or too big for you right now. You may be surrounded by clutter that you don't know what to do with. You could have piles of laundry that need to be taken care of. You may be in a place where these things seem like mountains to overcome. Just the simple act of taking care of yourself may seem overwhelming and too much effort.

Just keep traveling on this journey. One day, something is going to click for you. Some person or event will serve as a catalyst for you to make the changes you really want, but feel now like you cannot touch. The important thing is that you do have a desire to feel better. Keep at it. You will!

You may want to consider having your physician or psychiatrist put you on an anti-depressant for a time period. If you are like me, you may not want to do this. However, if you are at risk of harming yourself or falling in a deep abyss that you have a hard time coming out of, it may be very beneficial for a period of time. You do not have to stay on it forever. Speak with your physician about this and ask them about any risks associated with what they would prescribe. Having this as a booster in the background may allow you to begin to make the changes that a part of you is so desperately seeking.

Another reason to consider consulting with a qualified professional, like a psychiatrist, is that you want to find out if you have something causing anxiety or depression. Often, there is an underlying cause which can make it hard for you to bypass on your own. As serious as both of these conditions can be to your mental health, happiness and ability to function in your world, it is worth consulting with a doctor.

Holistic Helpers

The essence of the Yellow Mustard Flower (Sinapis arvensis) is great for helping to relieve depression. Other flower essences that also work well for this include:

- ❖ Blackberry
- ❖ Dill
- ❖ Borage
- ❖ Nectarine
- ❖ Sugar Beet
- ❖ Hellebore (black)
- ❖ Skullcap

Consider Elm (Ulmus procera) flower essence which is beneficial for anxiety or feeling you cannot cope well. Another one that works well if you are feeling like things are very dire is Gorse (Ulex europaeus). Other flower essences for anxiety include:

- ❖ Bells of Ireland
- ❖ Bottlebrush
- ❖ Forget Me Not
- ❖ Khat
- ❖ Prickly Pear Cactus
- ❖ Skullcap

❖ Sweet Flag

If you are feeling weak or unable to hold yourself together emotionally, Vine (Vitis vinifera) is a good flower essence to utilize. Dandelion flower essence brings calm and assists in releasing tensions held from overactive mental activity.

Gemstones To Assist in Calming Emotions

Watermelon Tourmaline is a remarkable stone that helps to cool and soothe emotions. Just like watermelon, it has a cool, calming effect. Emotional wounds we carry are greatly helped with this gem. Since it works directly on the heart area including that fourth chakra, it is beneficial to wear it as a necklace that extends into that region.

Smoky Quartz Crystal is primarily a grounding stone that has the capacity to diffuse negative energies. It is a natural choice for those with mood swings, who feel stressed or depressed.

Lepidolite is chosen by many who suffer from bi-polar disorder and depression. It can also calm those feeling considerable anxiety. When you are going through big changes, this is an excellent stone to wear or carry.

Tiger's Eye is an excellent stone for those suffering from anxiety. This gem assists with clear thinking so that you can resolve things in an easier manner. If you need extra willpower, this is a great choice.

The Sunstone Crystal is aptly named. With its shades of gold and orange, this is a stone that projects sunshine. It is very beneficial for depressed states and those affected by Seasonal Affective Disorder (SAD).

Rose Quartz Crystal is a favorite of mine for many reasons. First, it can be found easily and is not that expensive. Second, it serves so many different purposes — especially assisting us with self love. It has the capacity to help transmute negative energy into positive, making it uplifting to the spirit. This stone is soothing to the senses and a small stone kept in your pocket to rub your fingers over from time to time has a very calming effect. This beautiful pink crystal will also help you build your self esteem and worth.

Color Therapy can be a creative, fun way to relieve anxiety or depression. Whether you paint walls or canvas, this is a super way to change your mood and lift your spirit. If paint is not an option, doodle or color.

Music has the power to change the entire atmosphere of a vehicle, building, room and you! Experiment with listening to different types of music which are uplifting, relaxing and positive in nature. Try to avoid musical compilations that focus on lost love and hard times.

Lastly, the use of affirmations can be powerful short and long-term. When I began my healing, I listened to affirmations and positive material almost daily. It really helped to frame my day better and eventually retrain my mind to think, feel and believe differently. This was in the 1980's and I experienced limited audio choices. I would have to find and purchase cassette tapes and listen on my handy dandy Sony Walkman or in my car. Now, there are so many choices to choose from in our world. We can access so much through the Internet and quickly download an mp3.

In the next chapter, we will visit methods that can assist in curbing depression and anxiety.

Notes To Self

5 - Your Voice

Another critical step for healing is to speak to the right people about your abuse. Ideally, find a compassion based therapist. It could be a very dear friend. Truly, it needs to be someone you can trust your life with. Because as you begin to open up about your abuse, you will experience periods of deep relief, moments of great sorrow, and instances of hot anger. In other words, your emotions will fluctuate as things come to the surface. Do not be afraid of this. Take it very slow and go about things as it feels comfortable for you. Shining this light on the dark secrets you have held is critical. Having a pro there to guide you is very beneficial and you deserve nothing less.

It takes incredible courage to leave denial and share our secrets even with one person. To purchase the ticket for admission to healing, there is a cost. It is the price of letting go of your secrets and doing that safely with the right person or people.

Secrets like this are strange in the way they have the capacity to expand inside us. We may think we have tucked them away like a note in our pocket. Yet, the secrets take on an individual life of their own and grow in the dark as if they are a fungus inside. We really don't see this happening, yet these same secrets we have denied begin to scream for attention. It manifests as depression, anxiety, post traumatic stress, hypersexuality or hyposexuality. It affects our self-esteem. Letting go of our secrets is the first step to becoming who we could be versus who we feel we are.

In our world today, many do not want to read or hear about sexual abuse. However, this is changing. From the #metoo movement to people disclosing their abuse during a Ted Talk, the word is moving out and people are listening. Truly, we need to give that hurt part of you a voice and not continue to smash it. When you decide you will no longer ignore it, say it does not bother or affect you, things begin to shift and change. By living true and authentic, you set your spirit free to become something greater — perhaps something you never imagined before. Let us explore ways you may feel safe giving voice to that part of you that was wronged --- whether it happened fifty years, five years or two weeks ago.

When you make your voice heard, what you are essentially achieving is the acknowledgement and release of feelings. Each time you let out a little more of what was pushed deep inside and ignored, you heal a little. I happen to believe that feelings are all we really have in this world. We have our actions and things we have accomplished or achieved, but feelings were at the base of that or we would never have wanted to do it. Feelings are what I believe we take with us when we leave this earth - they are tied up with our memories. Indeed the feelings we hold inside make up who we are. How can you explore and reach those feelings that lack the attention and care they need in order for you to achieve healing? There are many modalities and this first one is one of the most crucial. Warning: many of you won't like hearing it; some of you have already been doing it and know what I say is true.

Yes, here it comes --- journaling. I know - many do not want to do it; makes excuses of why there is no time for such a thing; or too tired to do it. Really, what is holding you back from this step? Could it be fear lies at the bottom of it? Every person I know on the healing journey has had to find some form of journaling. I cannot express to you how important this is. I also empathize if you do not follow through and do it. Because I was like that - yes me the writer. I was not into getting those thoughts out at all, much less being tied to having to journal.

One of the things that some abuse survivors do is stay super busy. I fell into that group. It's an avoidance technique wherein you load your life up with so many activities that you never really have that quiet alone time to reflect on yourself. Journaling equals loving yourself – it is healing in ways you cannot imagine. It often leads to other forms of expression as you feel free to vent all that ugliness that really needs to come out at some point.

My first journal page about my sexual abuse looked like chicken scratch and made no sense to anyone but me. It was written on a small notepad page – not some fancy journal I purchased although you could do that if you want. When I came across the chicken scratch page years later, I could see in the handwriting and the short staccato like sentences that the person who wrote it was hurting. She wanted to just put short words like in a bullet form but without the bullets. I could also feel her shame around some of the words she wrote. Guess what? That little chicken scratch page is one of the best things I've ever written. Not that any editor would praise it, but it was the beginning of my journey in facing the feelings and facts that I had denied for so long.

I know you are probably eager to know ways you can advance yourself to another level in life. You want to not feel so affected by the abuse you endured. You are on the right track because you are seeking. When you seek, you find. A mind frame is set up that allows this to happen on an intellectual, emotional and energetic level. You are to be congratulated for where you are at.

I know from my studies and experience that where you are headed is a place that a part of you already exists. Now this may sound confusing, but when you understand that time itself is an illusion, it all makes sense. That is why I keep calling this a journey. If you try just a little, you can visualize the you that is more open, free and not burdened so much by your past. It exists right at the end of the road of this trip we are on together. It is real and there. You are traveling toward it. Indeed, it is calling for you to come. For those of you who have been on the journey for awhile now, that ever expanding you is still calling you to things greater than you imagined you could be.

You began as a beautiful whole flower that was trampled upon and crushed by the weight of people who wanted to control and steal your energy. On this journey together, we will move toward not only thriving in the garden of life, but blooming so brilliantly that it strikes a chord of deep respect from others when viewed from afar. Does that mean those same types of others will not continue to try and steal your energy in some way? NO! They will continue, perhaps in other ways not related to sexual abuse. This energy dance is constantly going on between individuals. We all participate in it. However, you will learn to prevent this while your petals unfold and reach for the sun. Knowledge is power to keep you from being trampled in any fashion in the future. It all takes time and learning it in small doses that you can then actively apply to your current situation.

For those of us that are away from the abusers, may we count ourselves fortunate to be in a position to try and feel whole again without being subjected to additional abuse. This is our journey we are on toward a brighter life filled with unexpected gifts and a greater connection to our self and others.

Let me mention again. What happens if you do not participate in the process of healing? You will experience predominately one of two overarching themes in your life. Either you will turn that hurt against yourself in self-sabotaging ways or you will turn it against others. At times, you could appear to do both. But, primarily you will be one or the other – self harm or harming others.

You see, almost everyone who is out there committing the abuse upon people, whether it be verbal, physical or sexual, has never healed what happened to them. They are following their deep seated anger and control issues that push them to hurt others. So, we need to understand this. It does not mean they are excused from what they have done. It is just an underlying explanation of why people do some of the incredibly awful things they do.

Why should you be silent no more? The number one reason is to propel you toward your own healing. Right behind your own needs are the needs of others – those who have been victimized and those who will be but it has not happened yet. The more we keep the conversation in the public domain and mainstream it, the more we can educate and protect others. Am I saying you need to get on television and proclaim your abuse? No, not at all. There are those who want to do this and should. You will not feel ready to be public until you have experienced quite a bit of healing. You may never want to go public or even tell friends or family (assuming they do not know).

Let's talk briefly about why you are trying to heal. In some way, you have an urge to feel better. You may also want to help others. You desire a life with meaning and purpose. Yet, you know in order to live that life, you have to get past your story and the ways it has thus far inhibited you.

While you are your story and that is a huge part of self identity, you are so much more. You know that because at times you have uncovered aspects of yourself that make you proud and give you confidence. This healing you have embarked on is a long road trip. Unfortunately, we do not have an option for the "beam me up Scottie" travel machine like an old episode of Star Trek. This is not a weekend seminar you are attending where you get all excited and "abracadabra", your life is fixed, only to find a week later that feeling wears off quickly. No, it's more like a road you are walking and sometimes, another friendly soul comes along and gives you a lift to the next town, helping you make faster progress. However, most of the time, you are moving yourself from point a to b – one step at a time.

Healing is work and it is not instant – although you can have some moments where you make a giant leap in the flash of a minute. I have experienced that at times and it does feel like it's been gifted to you. But, it will never happen if you fail to begin this work. Happiness is out there. You can do this. I and others are here for you.

When you first begin the trip, you realize you are completely overdressed. This starting point of your journey is the absolute most brutal. Your body is covered in many layers of coats and jackets. Each time you walk, sweat and make more headway on your trip, you take off one of those coats or jackets and toss it aside, lightening your load. You want to be free of this heavy feeling that you have been carrying around. You want to be light as a feather at times so you could just fly. Yet, you know that you would then only be blown by the wind ... and you need more direction and choice on what happens in your life. There is a part of you that knows you still need help on your journey and are not ready to travel so lightly. You want to discover what is in the next town, who you may meet along the road. Just remember, you are shedding layers of yourself and becoming lighter and lighter as you progress. Part of losing the burden you carry is tied up in the denial and shame of those secrets. The secrets can destroy your spirit if you cannot release them safely to the right source.

The word journal is at the root of the word journey. To journal is to keep a record (sometimes daily) of where you started, what transpired and where you ended. To journal is to keep track of your journey. For your purpose, to journal is to begin the release of things that you want to heal. You do not need to have anything new or fancy to write in. It can be a stack of paper; a small notebook;

anything you want or have available. The important thing is to just write. Write about anything and do not worry about the neatness of your handwriting, grammar or even making sentences correctly. This is for you. It can be a few single words at a time. Journaling does not take a lot of time. In fact, it can be done in ten or fifteen minutes. You can choose to do it daily or weekly. It might be helpful to find what times work best for you and then put a reminder on your phone or another calendar system to prompt you to write.

The Diary of Anne Frank is one of the most read books in the world, holding second place behind *The Holy Bible*. In this harrowing recount of her trials and tribulations, Anne showed us what faith and resilience look like in the face of extreme domination and danger. You have a story too. Let it unfold before you whether you begin with a few words, several paragraphs, or many pages. Let the tears flow. Allow your anger to come out on the pages. This is healing work you are engaged in. You do not have to limit yourself to writing words. Drawings can be more powerful than words. You could have a combination of both. There are no rules with this.

There was a Mexican artist named Frida Kahlo, who created a collection of poems, thoughts and colorful sketches in her journal. People describe it as a mixture of beautiful tragedy. She has since passed on to the greater life, but her journal was reprinted and made into a beautiful bound book with watercolor illustrations.

Journaling your journey in life does not have to become classic literature, a best seller or anything other than a tool that shows you where and how you need to heal the most. It is an escape valve for those feelings that have been bottled up inside for so long. Our feelings matter. We have been taught the reverse. Trust me when I tell you that your feelings really matter. When you address them with healing methods, you will be free to move forward in life toward greater self confidence, love, and prosperity.

I have cataloged many ways to accomplish this journal task without it being something you hate. Sign up at my website to download two free items that will assist you. One is a sheet with unique journal prompts to get you started and flowing. I also have a guided visualization in mp3 format you can lie down and listen to. This visualization is uniquely created to assist you in giving up your secrets. lyraadams.com

Holistic Helpers

To assist you in building your self-esteem, you may want to try the flower essence of Daffodil (*Narcissus ajax*). Another beneficial flower essence is African Marigold (*Tagetes erecta*).Still more that work well include Iris, Jasmine, American Paw Paw and Snapdragon.

Gemstones that are associated with the fifth chakra (throat area) of the body can be very beneficial for allowing you to speak your mind and use your voice to the right people. Almost all gems that help the throat chakra are blue in color. There are some exceptions. I am including some of the most popular, but there are many. For this 5th chakra area, you may want to try:

Blue Kyanite really encourages you to express yourself. So, if you are feeling stifled about speaking to others or even journaling, this would be a good stone to own.

Turquoise has many applications in healing and spiritual connection. One great benefit of this stone is it gives you confidence to speak your truth.

Lapis Lazuli is such a gorgeous blue color. It will assist in releasing things you felt too angry to talk about. Anytime you feel angry, reach for this stone.

Blue Lace Agate's appearance alone tells you that it soothes and calms. If you have said something harsh or if your words seem to come out wrong, this is a great stone to wear in the throat area. With time, this stone will assist wearers in communicating information, ideas and truths in the highest way possible as the gem is closely tied to the angelic realm.

Aquamarine is a wonderful stone that encourages honest communication. Some also find it gives them added courage to speak their truth.

Your Creative Voice

When you are limited on who you can speak to about your sexual abuse, it is very beneficial to explore ways to express your feelings through creative endeavors. You will find solace in the many ways possible to express your hurt and pain. Any expression of art is often an outlet for emotions. This could be anything from:

- Coloring
- Painting
- Writing
- Singing
- Dancing
- Playing instruments
- Making instruments
- Woodworking
- Cooking
- Knitting
- Crocheting
- Sewing
- Creating anything!

During these activities, we begin to engage the right side of our brains. We have a chance to express our feelings and put them into something that we call art. In art and creative pursuits, I find joy and am able to open myself to further inspiration. Other ideas to explore for creative expression are:

Body Movement – Most sexual abuse survivors disengage from their bodies and stay in their heads a lot. This keeps them from feeling grounded. I really recommend specific types of body movement that is grounding in nature. All forms of dance, yoga, qi gong and tai chi change your vibration and help create joy. They are all very beneficial.

Dreams – Our subconscious tries to work so many things out in our dreams. You could start a dream circle online for your friends where you talk about and analyze for one another. You can keep a dream journal just for yourself.

Blogging - You could begin a blog under a pen name writing about your experiences. This will not only use your creative voice, it will educate others. You can start a blog for free on Wordpress. They have paid plans also, but free is good.

Music - if you play an instrument, this is a great way to express feelings through the vibration of chords. If you sing, this is a further enhancement and uses your emotional expression in a number of ways physically.

By developing or continuing creative practices, you give yourself an emotional outlet for many of the things you do not feel safe relating in a more vocal way. Remember this when you feel thwarted and frustrated with your healing path. Often, dabbling in something different helps immensely. I found that the more I just threw myself into things I had an interest in exploring, the better I felt about myself. Participating in these types of activities allows us to learn more things and gives us confidence to go to that next level of healing and inspired living. Another thing that happens during creative pursuits and body work is that depression and anxiety magically go away – at least for a good period of time.

6 - On Auto-Pilot

When I was a young child, I spent many Sundays with my parents as they would drive around looking at homes. There was a building boom going on and my father had secured a good position as an engineer. They were saving to make the homeownership dream a reality and this involved shopping around quite a bit. One house we visited was locked and my parents attempted to peer in the windows. I followed their cue, but being much smaller in stature, put my hand on a wasp nest built under a brick window ledge. I was trying to hoist myself up so I could see inside too. Immediately, I was stung on the face multiple times. Everything after that is a blur to my memory. I don't remember riding back to our apartment. I just remember my mother slathering baking soda on my face the next day which was abnormally swollen with multiple stings. I wondered if I would have a normal face after the attack.

Now, you would think I would be deathly afraid of wasps, but I'm not. Don't get me wrong. I will not invite their presence, but they do not freak me out. Instead, I sort of feel nonchalant about them. I had to really think about this as I saw one in the room with me today as I was writing. How did I develop this attitude? I live with people that have never been stung by a wasp. However, as soon as they see one they are like, OMG! There's a wasp. Somebody do something!

I remember someone telling me (not sure who) that if you become frightened around such creatures it sends out a signal to them and they will possibly come after you. They told me to be still if one lands on you and the same for the bee. If you jerk or move and they feel your fear signals, they may sting. So, somewhere along the line, I adopted this stance with stinging creatures and it seems to serve me fine so far.

Certainly, I could have held onto the trauma I endured from the seven wasp stings on the face as a small child. I think for a time, I did. Yet when someone told me how I could keep it from happening — how I could control the situation when I saw one or if they landed on me, it changed from thereon.

This shows us that we can change how we perceive things we find threatening. It also shows how we can be in control of some outcomes by adjusting our reactions and behaviors. When it comes to people who may be predatory toward us, there are some instances where a change in our behavior or choices can avoid conflict with them. There are many instances where that would not work because you did not have prior knowledge that you were being stalked or about to be made a victim. So, each situation is different.

I bring up the wasp story only because we have so many buried memories that haunt us from our sexual transgressions that have happened. It could be as slight as a particular scent or the way someone walks or talks may trigger anxiety or a feeling of doom. Particular songs or sounds could haunt us. With retraining, we can learn to differentiate and know if something is really a threat or not and, if so, how we can minimize or eliminate that threat.

Let us explore those invisible, negative unnamed monsters that creep up at times for survivors of abuse. They pop up in strange ways at unpredictable times. You always know they are making their presence known because suddenly, you feel a sense of panic, fear, depression or lack of confidence to be able to handle things on your own. During these times, it is always good if you can call someone that understands and can talk you through it. Some survivors post on social media groups asking for help. But, what if you cannot do that … or do not want to do that? What if those methods are not working right now? Maybe you feel like you have tapped out that friend with this same old scenario too many times.

Many people unaffected by severe trauma do not understand how triggering can occur. The abuse memories are stored in a vault of our mind not always easily accessible. Certain sounds, scents, touch or even happenings can release some of the contents of the vault. At that time, a full memory of an event may occur. Often, a set of uncomfortable feelings arise that may not be easily identified.

The first thing you need to do when these feelings and little mind gremlins attack is to take a mental inventory. We must determine are you physically safe right now? Logically, if you are in a safe place, you have to ask yourself if there is anything really endangering you right now in this moment. If so, get help immediately. If not, try to work through it.

Most of the time, this is a memory feeling coming up from somewhere inside you that creates this. It is just a memory that made a huge impact on you in the past, nothing more. This memory could be making itself known because it wants to be remedied, healed within you. Instead of resisting that it is there and trying to deny it, go ahead and acknowledge it.

The first method I want to share is something you can do any place at any time. It can help with panic attacks, sudden fear and other symptoms of post traumatic stress. However, it can also work well for particular feelings you are experiencing such as being very anxious, nervous, sad or depressed.

You will need to use your imagination a bit. Breathe easily and fully during this exercise. In your mind, try to compartmentalize this memory feeling as if you could hold it at bay from your body – hold it in your hand in a bubble. Talk to it and tell it that you know it exists but what it represents does not reflect what is really going on right now. Tell the memory bubble that it is time for it to go because it is nothing but a remnant from the past. Firmly state to the memory bubble with emotion: "I live in the now."

Bring yourself into this now moment, recognizing that you can hold this memory feeling in its present form of a bubble in the palm of your hand. Then, just as you did as a child, blow the bubble away from you. In your mind, watch it float away from you and eventually pop becoming nothing, disappearing entirely. This fast exercise can really work well. It may take a few practice times. When you have a feeling memory appear, you can visualize it as another bubble – one that you have control over, can let go of and see disappear.

This next tool is more of a little homework project. Hopefully, it is something you will find fun. I was inspired to create it from several sources that I have seen do something similar for their own lives, but more toward their spiritual practice. But for our purpose, this project and process is for healing trauma symptoms of all types.

Create an area that is just your spot on the planet – your safe spot. The size of this spot can be tiny, small or large. It can be something in a corner, on a large table or desk, or take up quite a bit of a room. Make it the size that fits your desire and space available. Transform your chosen area into a shrine of all you love, find comfort in and brings you joy. Utilize a small table or stool in the corner of your room or beside your bed. You may want to begin with a piece of cloth as a table cover in a color or design that pleases you. If you do not have that, no worries. Place items in this area that make you feel happy or joyful.

Items to consider are a photo of someone you really enjoy and love. It could even be a picture of you – perhaps as a child, teen or later in life. We definitely need to be working on loving you too. Place a vase with your favorite flower. This could be a fresh flower that you replace every so often or a silk one you can easily obtain at so many different stores. Add something that smells good, whether it be your favorite cologne, perfume, incense, scented candle or other aromatherapy products.

Place something that connects you with your spiritual or religious faith, if any. This could be images of the Buddha, Jesus Christ, Mother Mary, an angel, Goddess archetypes -- whatever is appropriate for you. If you do not subscribe to anything like this, consider a beautiful landscape photo from a place you have visited or would like to visit. You might place a picture of your favorite super hero – one that you feel closely identified with and would be if you could. Any archetype you feel drawn to will work.

You may want to add a physical book --- one that you know you can open anywhere within it and read something valuable. I would have a notebook and pen available too. Add something soft you can hold if you want, or just stroke with your hand when you are out of sorts. This could be a small stuffed animal, a folded baby blanket you have kept since childhood, anything plush or soft that calls to your heart. And speaking of hearts, place an image of that on your table as well. How about a favorite rock, crystal, gemstone, sea shell or even a piece of jewelry that brings you joy?

Come up with your own ideas which I am sure will resonate with you stronger. This sacred area must be about you and what brings you feelings of contentment. You might want to place a soft rug in front of this area for your comfort when sitting. If you prefer sitting in a chair, maybe you have room to place it beside your special area.

Now, what is the point of this little shrine? It represents all that you love, trust and find joy in. It is also a physical place that you can touch and go to when you need to transcend what you are feeling and be "in the now". This is your sacred space. It is an area that holds special meaning just for you and you only.

When you feel fearful or are experiencing any distressed feelings, go to your shrine. If possible, sit cross legged on the floor in front of your joy area. Touch and hold your items. Journal any thoughts you have at this time or speak them into a recorder on your phone.

Breathe! Through your nose, take deep, but comfortable, breaths that expand your belly. Allow the air to blow out your mouth. In through the nose – out through the mouth. As you exhale, see all negativity in your mind's eye leaving your body. Do this several times.

If possible, play soft relaxing music that assists you in calming your inner self.

Repeat in your mind: "All is well. Everything will work out for me. I may not have all the answers now, but they are coming. All is well with me."

All survivors of any type of trauma can benefit from this simple, yet effective, way of helping to dissolve the internal conflicts that can arise from time to time. When we practice this method, we put ourselves into the now. It is a mindfulness practice that brings us back into our body, grounds us and helps us to feel safe and collected again.

This practice will assist people who have endured any type of abuse, not just sexual. It will assist those who have post traumatic stress, anxiety, depression, panic attacks and fears that crop up unpredictably at the sound of a noise or some other triggering event.

If you truly have no room for it because you live in a New York City apartment-sized place, use a small decorative box, trunk or suitcase to house your special items? That way, you can pull it out when needed.

If you travel in your vehicle frequently, you can set up a mini version of your shrine there as well. If you suffer a panic attack while driving, simply pull off the road and duplicate what you would do at your home shrine as much as possible.

As you put this into practice for yourself and actually utilize it when feeling out of sorts, you will begin to retrain your brain. You will find solace and peace in the simple pleasures surrounding you. It is an act of kindness and compassion to engage in this activity for you. Stay calm, breathe and know that you may not have all answers, but all is well and will be even better soon.

When the wasp lands on my arm, I slowly breathe, center and stay calm. All is well with me and it leaves. Our trauma memories can be dealt with in a similar manner. Try to stay calm with slow deep breathing. Center yourself with items that make you feel safe and loved. Treat yourself with loving self care. This builds your armor — your thick coating on your petals where eventually these items will not bother you as much. If you fail at first and still feel great emotions, this is fine. Be patient with yourself — loving with you. Own the fact that you are trying and will continue to try; knowing you will be better with each attempt.

Notes To Self

7 - Feeling Comfortable In Your Skin

Recently, I randomly chose two fictional books to listen to on audio. Unknowingly, each of these books had a very similar theme although the story lines were quite different. I felt it was another synchronistic event that I had come across these two books back to back. The subject matter dealt with the question we must ask ourselves at times: How comfortable are we in our skin given the abuse we have endured?

The first book I chose was called *Where the Forest Meets the Stars* by Glendy Vanderah. In the story, a young girl still wearing her pajamas shows up in an unlikely place -- a forested small community. When questioned, she claims she is from another planet. While there is some humor in her responses to the inquiries from adults she encounters, her answers hide a mystery that unfolds throughout the book. There was a scene toward the end that did trigger me somewhat but not too bad. I don't want to tell you much more except that if you want to dig into some fiction it is an excellent choice.

The second book I randomly chose had similar themes. The title of this one is *When We Believed in Mermaids* by Barbara O'Neal. This is the story of two sisters who are separated by the supposed death of the older one. Fifteen years after this faux death, the sister is spotted briefly on a television newscast by her mother and younger sister. The entire time you are reading or listening to the book, you are wondering why this sister would fake her death and create an entire new identity – in fact, becoming a different person to a large degree. Again, there is a very similar concept with identity crisis in this book. Toward the last third of the book, you begin to understand why the older sister wanted to kill off the old self and become someone new.

For much of my life, I wanted to be someone other than the person that I was. This started at a very young age. Once my sexual abuse happened, the shame I carried solidified my desire to be anyone other than who I was.

Many times in the field of psychology, we hear of those who experience a real crisis of identity, also known as dissociation. There are several definitions of dissociation in the psychological literature. For this conversation, we are going to be using the one that closely aligns with our particular life experiences. This definition was put forth by Dr. Marlene Steinberg and author, Maxine Schnall (Steinberg & Schnall, 2001). Briefly, they defined dissociation as:

> "an adaptive defense in response to high stress or trauma characterized by memory loss and a sense of disconnection from oneself or one's surroundings."

This could be experienced many different ways. One could have a black out period with their memory – something that is not induced with drugs or alcohol, but a true gap of memory for a period of time. Another way one could experience dissociation is by blocking pain or pleasure sensations in the body which is often accompanied by a shutting down of emotional responses as well. In some cases, dissociation can develop into other alter personalities that make us feel more comfortable or capable in some way. What begins as a natural human response to painful events can lead to this.

Dissociation can be a shutting off or closing down of emotions. It can be gaps in memory so that we do not have to know what actually happened. It can be a blocking of physical sensations such as pain and/or pleasure, making it difficult for us to be real with ourselves and what our responses could be in relationships and other situations. It can be the feeling of wanting to be someone other than our real selves. It can be a self loathing or hatred for the real self. It can also be confusion about who we really are (Pollock, 2015).

All of these are ways we can dissociate from trauma we have experienced. It begins at the time of the trauma or shortly thereafter. It is a natural human reaction that is protective in nature. It only becomes an issue for us if it carries over well after the trauma has ended and follows us in life. Left untreated, it can easily be triggered by stress we feel in everyday life. Even though the stressful event we are experiencing is not related to the abuse we endured, it has now become part of a learned response.

One of the great things about practicing being "in the now" is that it assists us in staying grounded and not slipping into any type of dissociation. During trauma, dissociation served a purpose in protecting our minds. Now, it could be more of a hindrance to our joyful development in life.

In my lay opinion, dissociation is just a method of slipping out of your current "now" reality. When it is associated with traumatic events, it can be a valuable escape hatch for us – a way to psychologically survive. This can occur to a mild degree or in a major way. If you are a student in a class you consider boring, you may find yourself allowing your mind to daydream. You will not remember anything your professor said during this time. This would be a very mild way of dissociating from your current reality. Basically, disassociation is a mechanism kicking in for us to disconnect … something that allows us to put our mind in one place while our body stays in its physical location.

In today's psychology community, dissociation and its associated disorders that can occur are still being precisely defined. Much advancement has been made in this area. There is debate on not only the way it occurs in humans, but also a clear definition. I would propose this could be due to the fact that we all react differently to things. To a degree, it is stigmatized by some. We have people who hardly believe in it and at the other extreme those who see it as a full-blown phenomenon that occurs.

Dissociative Identity Disorder is the new name for multiple personality disorder. We may hear someone declare, "Oh, she was abused and she dissociated, leaving her body. Afterward, she turned into a Sybil-like character with 21 different personalities." This is the extreme and when we use the word dissociation, some people see this type of definition in their mind. Splitting of the ego and different personalities appearing can and does happen to some. However, there are many in-between scenarios.

When we are speaking of it as a disorder, it seems to be in response to extreme overwhelmed feelings induced by traumatic events. And while it was handy to experience dissociation during the trauma, it can become a coping habit in the future from anything we want to avoid. This is because the escape method is locked into the brain as a pattern of avoidance. You may feel that trauma is about to or is occurring again from some outside trigger. This is the point where it is disordered in your system and needs correction.

There are many events that could lead to ongoing dissociation disorders. Before I list some of them, I also want to stress that you may have experienced dissociation with your trauma at the time, but have not had it return in your life. If that is the case, you are not operating in a disordered way. Some of the events that can cause dissociation are childhood neglect, abuse, sexual abuse as child, adolescent or adult, a bad accident, war, being a victim of a violent crime such as a robbery, a natural disaster, prisoner of war or torture, sex trafficking, mind programming, ritual abuse, repeated medical procedures especially if pain is involved, and witnessing genocide. Any of those hellish conditions have the capacity to leave a residue behind. We see this often with post traumatic stress disorder (PTSD) which is linked to trauma. But we also see it with people who try not to feel.

Several studies show that higher scores of dissociation are linked to higher rates of depression and suicide. These higher scores also include increased rates of substance and alcohol abuse, self injury, smoking and other self destructive behaviors. To know if we are still experiencing dissociation and it has turned into a disordered pattern for us, we can look at the following symptoms of which you may have one or more. To know for sure, consult a qualified psychologist or psychiatrist. The current DSM-V lists symptoms and severity of those.

> Amnesia can be a symptom. This would be akin to black-out periods of time you cannot remember except that there is no cause from alcohol or drugs.
> Depersonalization is another symptom in which you may feel detached from your emotions, yourself in general, or even parts of your body. You may feel robotic like you just go through the motions.
> Derealization is the third symptom in which a person may feel totally detached from other people and their surroundings. They may have thoughts or feelings that the world around them is not real.
> Identity Confusion is the fourth symptom where a person might have real questions and conflict about who they are.
> The last symptom is Identity Alteration. With this symptom, there would be actual

personality differences that other people who know you really notice. For the person experiencing this, there may be a feeling that they cannot control these new identities. This last symptom falls close to what we hear of as multiple personality disorder (American Psychiatric Association, 2013).

Overall, we are looking to numb ourselves from pain. Did you know that many, if not most, sexual abuse victims find themselves almost in a state of being frozen when the event occurs? The feeling that overtakes them is like a deer staring at the headlights of an oncoming vehicle. Many survivors beat up on themselves because they were not one of the ones that "fought back". This blame is so misplaced. You see, it all comes down to the systems of the body – specifically the autonomic and parasympathetic systems.

In the autonomic, you have your fight or flight syndrome and people are generally geared one way or the other. On a biological level, I see it as being beyond adrenal and cortisol hormonal reactions. It could be connected to the vagus nerve which has many different tasks in our body. This is something not completely known. No matter how it occurs, there is a consistent splitting of reality wherein the mind takes us on a little detour away from the reality we so want to escape. This often includes traumatic events where we feel we have no control. So this is something to consider because there are those who say they must have not really been raped because they did not fight back. They can become confused believing it to be consensual in some way because they did not fight hard enough. Often, fear and coercion are involved on the perpetrator's end to control the victim of abuse.

This is a phenomenon much like when an animal freezes or feigns death to keep a predator from attacking. Often, if fight or flight feels more risky, this coping mechanism of being still, freezing and not fleeing or fighting takes over. This can even produce actual fainting and more often, a sort of trance state wherein the victim is coping in this manner. There can even be a heightened insensitivity during this time to pain in order to protect one's self. Some victims report feeling as if their mind split in two – part of them was present in that moment and part of them was somewhere else mentally. In other words, the victim's parasympathetic nervous system is producing this behavior as a protection mechanism to not experience the event or pain associated with it. It's a mental checking out. I know that I experienced this. Specifically, I experienced dissociative amnesia in which I do not remember parts of what occurred to me during the time I was with my abuser. I have found that some things did come back to me in bits and pieces.

Another way of experiencing dissociation is feeling as if you are not in this world. Some may feel they are not in their own body. Generally, this often happens to victims during abuse – as if they are watching what is happening, but not part of it. If this is ongoing for you, it is possible you are experiencing what professionals have identified as depersonalization disorder.

How can a person know if they have experienced dissociation? For me, it was having memory flashbacks of things that happened that I did not remember before. As I examined this, I realized there were other periods of time, both short and long, that I had no memory of what went on. To protect my psyche, I checked out into another state of consciousness. Again, it's just like when you are driving home and lose yourself. When you arrive, you realize that you do not remember passing certain common landmarks or whether you stopped for any red lights. This auto-pilot persona we slip into is a glimpse into what full dissociation can be.

This disorder can also affect your identity. This is what used to be called multiple personality disorder. Now it is referred to as Dissociative Identity Disorder. This is where you experience at least two distinct personalities that have different ways of behaving, thinking and even separate memories. Clues that you may be experiencing this would be memory lapses in your current ordinary life. Dissociation is not always about having multiple personalities, but it can be. If you suspect you may be experiencing this, consult with a professional to assess what may be going on so you can know what you are experiencing for sure or not. All symptoms of dissociation are manageable with therapeutic techniques, so you should not be alarmed of any indications you may have noticed about yourself. The fact that you are aware and want to know is a huge portion of healing any condition that exists.

If you know or suspect that you have experienced dissociation disorder at the time of your trauma or any other time in life, here is an interesting side note. You may do it again, especially during periods of stress. Since it has been relied upon in the past as a coping mechanism, it may be unintentionally used again. This is especially true if this happened to you during childhood. Your brain and personality are still forming then and this may be a grooved pattern in your long playing record that allows you to cope by pretending things are happening outside of yourself and not to you.

As much as I would love to recommend a holistic practice to remedy any current dissociation or depersonalization disorder, the choices are limited. Living in the now — being in the now is one of the best holistic practices for bringing your conscious awareness back into your body. Working with your shrine I spoke of previously and grounding your body through relaxation and breathing is important as well. Our first chakra at the base of our torso deals with feelings of survival, safety and fear. We will be focusing on each of the chakras in chapter 14.

Another helpful holistic approach spoke of later in this book is inner child and trauma wound healing. In that section, we will focus upon healing the inner child within us. This work is very important. One reason is many of us, as survivors, feel that if people really knew everything about us, they would not like us. There are many survivors who have trouble liking themselves. By going back and working with the inner child or adolescent, we begin to reveal who we are at a core level – the real us – the beautiful soul that was born into this world innocent, perfect, and with a wonderful purpose that can unfold if it is given the right environment.

Flower essences for coping with life and crisis of identity include four leaf clover, banana, henna, mallow, papaya, American paw paw, pimpernel and squash.

I recommend that all survivors explore the depths of denial they may be diving into along with any possible dissociation that could be happening with a licensed professional therapist. Things that are not dealt with can lead to depression and suicidal thoughts. You could feel like harming yourself or someone else. So, it is really important to pick up the phone and make an appointment. You cannot rely on joining a social media group to get your advice on more complex issues. While you may receive some opinions (and that is all they are) that help, ultimately, you need to talk with a trained compassionate professional who can assist you.

I want you to know that almost everything I speak to you about I have struggled with myself. There are times when healing can feel like such a tremendous amount of work. I remember being very overwhelmed at times and discouraged, wondering if I would get my life straightened out. I wondered if I would feel more "normal" in social settings and different circumstances. Basically, would I feel good about myself finally? It takes time, but it can and does happen. But, I have learned that healing unfolds in layers just like the lotus flower. When you believe you have done the work to heal abuse and made such headway, things can and will challenge you to dig deeper and go farther to unfold even more. And this is a beautiful thing to have happen. It is not something to fear.

8 - Taming The Dragon

You're walking alone at dusk. You hear footsteps in the distance behind you. Immediately, your mind begins to sort out if this could be danger. You try to talk yourself down. "It's alright, nothing to be afraid of. -- just another person walking and it does not mean they are following me". But fear comes in a sharper way. Your heart rate increases exponentially. Should you turn to see who it is? Should you run? Finally, you gather courage to turn around and see the person following you approaching a vehicle on the street and getting inside. "It was nothing. Thank God it was nothing." This is a common example – very common – of what happens to people suffering from post traumatic stress.

Trauma touches all of us in some way. Basically, no one escapes it and it takes many forms. Personal trauma can occur with events that affect many people such as war, famines, earthquakes and floods. Trauma can occur from accidents or sudden physical attacks. It can be experienced with divorce or losing a beloved relative or pet. Trauma certainly happens with emotional, physical or sexual abuse.

But, what is trauma exactly? There are several definitions but I think one that succinctly sums it up is that trauma is the psychological and emotional response to very stressful events. And I want to add that these are things that hurt the person involved in some way whether it is physically, psychologically or even spiritually. This event or events would be something you initially want to deny is happening. Often, denial is the first response. Depending on the level of the trauma, you may also experience a period of shock. Very often, you hear survivors of trauma say that it felt surreal – as if it was not really happening – except that it was.

There are different levels of trauma. In the instance of a onetime event such as a single rape or seeing someone murdered, you would experience what is termed acute trauma. If you have been subjected to trauma over a period of time, this would be classified as chronic trauma. This often occurs with long term abuse of any type. Complex trauma is the third type identified in the field of psychology. It is described as the person traumatized having been subjected to multiple events that are varied and traumatic in nature.

I want to paraphrase from my book, *Dreaming Synchronicity*, how I came to look at trauma. First, as I said at the beginning: everyone is going to experience some form of it during their life. Second, trauma will try to own us. I see it as a pet dragon we carry in our pocket that can rise up at times, breathing fire and unleashing a fury. Yet, I have learned over time that even though that pet dragon stays with us, we have the power to subdue it.

Just as there are the three main levels of trauma, there are at least five main levels of PTSD. I am going to focus on Complex Post Traumatic Stress Disorder or C-PTSD in this writing. Personal identity can be affected by the abuse we endured. This is a pervasive situation with survivors of all abuse. Confusion or loss of identity is a common component of C-PTSD or Complex Post Traumatic Stress Disorder. I believe it is possible that many abuse survivors experience C-PTSD and do so until they effectively work it out for themselves with qualified therapy or other healing modalities.

One of the strangest aspects of this condition is that you really may be going through life not knowing you are experiencing it. Instead of actual flashbacks to events of your past that were abusive in nature, you might find that you have trouble with relationships, jobs and keep choosing the wrong kind of partner. And, this is not to say that particular things may not still trigger you. There could be certain subjects discussed or events happen during a movie you are watching that bring on a feeling of panic. This can very well happen. But, for the most part, you may find that you do not experience flashbacks so much as you are struggling to have a great life.

Everyone assumes flashbacks happen. It is true this can occur. Yet, it is more likely that you may experience the same emotions you felt when your abuse occurred. This emotional flashback can leave you feeling unable to work and cope as you normally do in your life. It can color your entire experience of life keeping you from your good. While usually temporary in nature, flashbacks of any type signal work you need to do. So, it is important to seek a professional who can assist you with this.

Have you seen movies where the space crew comes back into earth's orbit or the military personnel return from a clandestine mission? The first thing that happens is they enter a debriefing. Now, what exactly happens there in those instances, we do not know. However, a trained professional can help you unpack and debrief the traumatic events of your life. They can give you tools that assist you in coping and getting on to the better life you deserve. It takes time. You won't be there for just one hour and it is done. Instead, you will need to participate in your debriefing or recovery over time. Most of the work will be accomplished on your own, but having the pro there to coach and assist you is paramount.

Some people will tell you that Complex PTSD is permanent with no cure. I disagree. I think that we will always carry our memories like that little dragon in our pocket. Yet, we can rise above many of the destructive patterns and problems that occur in our lives. We also can learn tools to cope and thrive instead of allowing the dragon to rule us. So, do not listen to people --- and I mean that even for professionals – who say something is incurable. It may be chronic, but it can be managed very effectively with the right approaches to healing. Grace and healing can occur without notice.

The causes of C-PTSD are many. It can come from viewing or being directly involved in domestic violence or abuse, especially if this happened repeatedly. It can come from being neglected or abandoned as a child by one or both parents. Certainly, it can occur from verbal, physical, emotional and sexual abuse at any age. Yet, the younger it occurs, the more complex it may be. If you have been a prisoner of war, tortured, kidnapped, held in human bondage it can happen. If you were trafficked by others, it definitely can happen. How do we know if we are suffering in such a way that it is affecting our identity? Here are some clues:

- ❖ You may feel very separate from others--- like there is a defective difference you carry and others do not. This creates feelings of isolation.
- ❖ In addition, you may feel that no one understands or can really comprehend your experiences.
- ❖ You may be highly self critical
- ❖ Self worth is often low with Complex PTSD and there can be a very real self loathing along with thoughts of hurting yourself or suicide at times.
- ❖ You might feel intense anger for no logical reason.

There can be some trauma bonding between you and your main perpetrator. This would be where you feel like you need to minimize the effect this individual had upon you, rather than place the blame where it should lie. On the other hand, you may seek personal revenge upon your perpetrator.

Another symptom is having a difficult time trusting others – trusting just about anyone in fact. Lord knows this is a natural reaction, especially if you have been abused repeatedly as is often the case. But, even with some one-time events, you can find it difficult to walk into certain buildings or travel down particular streets. You may carry a fear to even fall asleep at night. All of this is a lack of trust that you will be okay.

Some individuals are misdiagnosed with borderline personality disorder because it shares some of the same symptoms as C-PTSD. You should be aware of this if any medical provider has diagnosed you with such and perhaps seek another opinion. Also be aware that if you have complex PTSD, you may still have some of the symptoms of regular PTSD. Therapies for the complex PTSD are still evolving to see what works for people and what does not. You may also engage in some therapies used for those who endure PTSD. Some of the newer treatments available include Eye Movement Desensitization and Reprocessing (EMDR). EMDR therapy is fascinating and holds the potential to speed healing much faster than traditional methods. To find out more about this method, visit EMDR.com

Today, there are also many practitioners who are experienced with compassionate trauma based therapy. This is something to inquire about and look for if you have a choice in the matter.

Listen to music during these stressful times that slow down your breathing and help sooth you.

I highly recommend the regular use of affirmations. I stress their use often to those on a healing journey because I know they work. It takes repetition as you are retraining your brain — laying down new neural pathways of messages that are life affirming and positive. Gradually, you will begin to see that you think and operate differently from repeating positive loving and life affirming statements.

Try to get into the habit of writing down your feelings – good and bad. A diary or journal of your thoughts and feelings is so beneficial to you. I still journal regularly, even if it is just to vent which is healthy too.

If you have limited funds or no insurance coverage for professional counseling, try joining a group of survivors close to your area where you meet up once a week or so. For those of you who have been through considerable counseling and work, do you recognize that you still could do more things to really take your life to the next great level? If so, be proactive and figure out what your next move should be to love yourself more and give yourself a chance at your best life.

Always reach out to others who understand about these subjects when you need advice or an ear to listen. Do not waste time speaking to those who cannot offer you the type of advice or direction you may need.

Above all, know that you are a beautiful being that has come to this place and time with a purpose. Discovery of self is your key to unlocking that information. I believe in you! If I could discover all of this, you can as well.

Feeling Safe & Competent

Have you ever wondered when you will finally feel safe and that some boogie man is not going to sneak attack you? Have you longed to feel a peaceful contentment that all is right in your world? Have you wondered what you can do to feel more competent and experience a true confidence about yourself?

Panic attacks or anxiety can occur for many years after your experience with those who have transgressed you. The trauma you endured can be triggered by the smallest of things as spoken of earlier. By working at methods of reframing, we can eliminate much of the post traumatic stress we encounter in our lives as we go about trying to continue toward a life that is whole and meaningful to us. The number one thing you can do for yourself is always look within. This must be accomplished in a non-judgmental, loving way. We should never blame ourselves. The blame for what happened lies solely with our transgressors.

When anxiety or full blown panic overcomes you, try to get centered into the "now". Be present in what is right around you. Attempt to change your focus by noticing the ground you are sitting or standing on. What does it consist of – grass, dirt, sand, rock, carpet, concrete, wood, tile? Just take a moment and think about what you stand or sit upon - put your focus there for a few moments. If you are outdoors or can be quickly, remove your shoes and feel the earth beneath your feet. Merge with it. This is an instant grounding technique that in a certain way keeps you from electrical overload.

Your body is electric. Your very heart depends upon this current to run day and night. Sometimes, our heads can be so busy thinking thoughts or drudging up partial or full memories from the past that it is literally interfering with our balance. If you cannot get outside due to inclement weather or some other physical constraint, attempt to put your feet in warm water and give yourself a foot bath. Take time to massage your toes and the soles of your feet. Dry and pat your feet. Water allows us to wash away many things that ail us. Bless the water as you do this, and thank it for carrying your worries away.

Suppose you are at work where you can do none of this and you are feeling very anxious or like a panic attack may occur, use your hands in the same manner. Perhaps excuse yourself to the bathroom. Put your hands in the warm water and imagine all worries being carried away.

Bless the water in the same manner as you imagine letting go of anything that feels negative at this moment.

Building Confidence through Competence

Another idea to assist you in feeling more safe ... especially those of you who have been attacked in a violent physical way or held captive, is to consider learning some type of self defense method. There are many classes you can attend where you will learn basic, intermediate and advanced techniques for handling situations where others want to control or hurt you. I really believe this is not talked about enough in the healing community. Being trained in self defense will not only make you feel more confident and strong, it will assist you in beginning to lose many of the sudden unknown fears that crop up from events held in your subconscious.

Once you know that you can handle particular situations with more finesse, your fear levels decrease. This does not mean they disappear entirely, but tend not to have the panic hold on you as they did before. Any type of self defense training could be beneficial for adding skills and building confidence. There are many forms of martial arts that do this. In addition to building skills in dealing with an attacker or intruder, they assist you in building a discipline around the entire mind and body which increases your life force.

If you are unable, due to physical disabilities, to engage in forms of physical self defense, you could consider weapons training. Some survivors may want to do both. I realize this is a topic that is controversial, but even knowing what you would do with a baseball bat, sword or knife could assist you in feeling more confident when you experience fear or an actual attack from someone. Most of the time, there is no one that is going to attack you. Rather, it is our fears coming up that make us think of the "what ifs".

What if that noise you heard outside your door at night is an intruder? What if that man that walks a certain way coming toward you at dusk down the city sidewalk tries to attack you? Most of what we feel is made up of "future what ifs" and are not actually what is going on "now" around us. This is why grounding yourself in the present moment (in the now) is important.

If you want to consider gun ownership for protection, get fully trained in how to use the weapon. Make sure you are mentally stable enough to own weapons in general. Go to classes and spend time regularly at a shooting range. You may want to install a security system where you live so that you can sleep with ease if that is an issue for you.

By taking action and doing something to build your competency to deal with a threatening situation, you will gain more confidence. It is most likely that your new skills will never be needed. However, this will give you some peace of mind to be more proactive if something were to occur.

Pine tree sap (Pinus sylvestris) is very cleansing and purifying in nature. It will help correct unhealthy thought patterns which could be helpful in many different applications, especially with memory feelings that crop up from time to time. The scent is strong as this is the sap and not a flower essence. Place a small drop of the resin in an aromatherapy burner for usage.

Mimulus (Mimulus guttatus) is an excellent flower essence for feeling safer and stronger. If you are suffering from a lot of flashbacks, memories or dark thoughts, use the flower essence of Cherry Plum (Prunus cerasifera).

Notes To Self

9 – Addictions

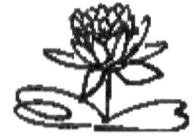

In this section, I want to briefly cover many of the most common addictions. While I will hit the main points of each, more information can be found individually on each addiction in numerous books and publications. At the end of this section, I will list holistic methods that may assist anyone suffering from addiction.

People with addictions are generally very creative individuals. They are also filled with deep feelings. Their addiction(s) assist them in subduing many of those emotions they find too overwhelming either in a positive or negative way. For instance, no matter what your poison is, you may feel compelled to partake of it when you are exceptionally happy, as much as when you are feeling something negative.

One flower essence that can assist with feelings and leveling things out is Manzanita (Arctostaphylos mansanita). If you need to be able to express your feelings better to others, Snapdragon (Antirrhinum majus) flower essence is a good one to try.

Many who have been affected by abuse carry addictions to something. Initially, an addiction is a way to avoid and numb our feelings. The means to do this is varied. All addictions take from us — they rob us of our life force. At the core of all addiction is an avoidance of our real self. It can begin that way because even for temporary moments, our anxiety or our usual way of being numbed is not present. Addiction also involves habits and the difficulty of change. When we hear the phrase we are creatures of habit, this is literal and very true. It takes concentrated effort and tremendous inside and outside resources to change something that has become a habit.

Ultimately, addictions produce conflict for us within our very being on physical, mental and spiritual levels.

We have been told there are psychologically addicting items and physical. Intuitively, I feel that we do not know everything there is to know about addiction and there could be many new things to discover about what is really physically needed or only psychological. For one thing, our medical system of the western world has separated psychological from physical in almost all instances of disorders and disease. Yet, they are interrelated. This is like saying your shoulder has no effect upon the use of your hand. They go together. Likewise, western medicine has ignored or forgotten the unseen component of the etheric body, chakra system and auric field. Thankfully, with the influence of holistic practitioners, this is changing with some traditional physicians and medical caregivers.

In my spiritual teachings, alcohol and drugs are said to make holes in the aura of an individual. This can lead to unwanted negative influences. On a metaphysical level, alcohol and drugs feel great because they expand this auric energetic bubble around you, making it larger. As it enlarges, holes or tears can occur. Your aura is like a protective film surrounding you that keeps negative entities and energies from slipping in and affecting you. These energies can be physical and non-physical. It often affects your boundary setting with other people. While many substances can be used to gain glimpses into other states of consciousness that exist, it should be used with caution and limited.

Have you ever felt hung over from partaking of a little too much mind altering substances? Your own physical vitality can be leaking from you within the auric damage. This is combined with actual physical damage, even if temporary. This is why you will want to rest afterward. This recovery period is needed.

Later in this book, I will mention other things that affect your physical and non-physical body ... or as I like to call it, your mind/body/spirit complex. For now, let's explore common things humans become addicted to.

Alcohol

Physically, addictions hurt the body in some way due to overuse and/or consumption. A glass of wine can be healthy for you from time to time. Yet, overuse of alcohol can create a long list of physical ailments. Did you know that hundreds of people in the United States die from alcohol poisoning each year? This is generally related to "binge drinking" (CDC, 2015). Binge drinking is defined as consuming large amounts of alcohol in a short period of time. This equates to 4 or more alcoholic drinks for women and 5 for men in a short period of time. It can cause the brain to shut down areas that control breathing, heart rate and more. Overall, alcohol related deaths in the United States are the third leading cause of death and it is all preventable. This would include vehicular accidents, heart problems, strokes, and many other medical conditions caused by alcoholism.

Short term effects can include:
- Vomiting
- Loss of critical thinking or judgment which could lead to further endangerment of self or others
- Loss of coordination
- Higher blood pressure
- Passing out and injury

Long term effects of alcohol abuse can include:
- Cardiomyopathy
- High Blood Pressure
- Stroke

- ❖ Irregular heart beat
- ❖ Alcoholic hepatitis.
- ❖ Liver fibrosis
- ❖ Fatty Liver
- ❖ Throat, mouth, larynx cancer
- ❖ Breast, liver, colorectal or esophageal cancer

Mental Effects of alcohol abuse can include:
- ❖ Learning Difficulties
- ❖ Loss of memory
- ❖ Easily confused
- ❖ Attention Span Challenges
- ❖ Actual diminished gray and white matter within the brain

That is very scary!

Alcohol affects some by serving as a depressant on the central nervous system. For others, it may actually stimulate activity. Many methods for healing sexual abuse require you to be as substance free as possible. Healing from the horrific tragedy you endured is serious work that can provoke some peak emotions at times. It will be important you are able to handle this in a sober manner to protect yourself from harm. If you use alcohol to excess, it truly can alter brain functions as well (Monico & Stein, 2020). Much of the healing that goes on emotionally on your journey will help lay down new neural pathways in your brain that are positive in nature. Alcohol and drugs can and will inhibit that process.

The flower essence of Angelica works well for alcoholism as well as the flower essence of Pennyroyal.

Food Addiction

Within different personalities lies the potential to use food as comfort for our emotions. In many cultures, including the United States, holidays and family times together center around food being prepared and available for all attending. Food is necessary. We need it to fuel our physical bodies.

Food can also be a very sensual experience as it involves touch, smell, taste and visual aspects. Let's face it; your favorite foods make you feel something. Chocolate has long been seen as a short substitute for love. The smell of fresh baked bread and many other food smells can make your mouth salivate. However, when we make food too close of a friend, it can actually work against us.

Within all food are chemicals that instantly begin working on our interior bodies as we ingest them. Some of the processes occurring inside of us are good and others not so good. Many starches turn almost instantly into sugars in our system. There are healthy, good fats and more toxic bad fats. Sugar is added to numerous processed foods along with salt.

While we need many of these substances for balance, too much of anything is not good for us and can lead to serious health consequences. If we gain a lot of weight, it can also affect us psychologically. There is a movement now for people that are overweight to be admired for their physiques as they are. There is nothing wrong with that at all. In fact, the healthiest thing you can do for yourself is to take off all your clothes, stand in front of a mirror and say with true meaning, "I love you and you are beautiful (handsome)".

Yet, I want to approach this section with the idea that sometimes we know we are absolutely addicted to something and we would fight for it. It will come before other things on our priority list of life. We must have it. At that point, it is an addiction.

Eric Clapton was once asked what the first drug was he became addicted to. He replied, "Sugar". It was a surprising answer and I assume Mr. Clapton was saying that this substance set up a desire in his brain for this type of stimulation. Sugar has the capacity to spike our blood that travels through our veins to our brains and tickle it in ways we find appealing — just like many drugs do. In other words, we get a real good feeling from that substance and our brain remembers it. It will want to continue experiencing that.

When you are addicted to food, you are essentially addicted to a pleasure cycle. Many things can set this up for an individual in their life including sexual abuse.

Physical dangers of food addictions include:

- Arthritis
- Chronic Pain
- Digestive Issues
- Diabetes
- Fatigue
- Headaches
- Heart Disease
- Kidney Disease
- Liver Disease
- Obesity
- Sexual Dysfunctions
- Sleep Issues
- Stroke
- And more …

Psychological factors for those affected by food addiction may include:

- Anxiety

- ❖ Depression
- ❖ Detachment from others
- ❖ Feeling Suicidal
- ❖ Low Self-esteem
- ❖ Panic Attacks

Those that have never suffered food addiction may believe that solving this issue is easy. In fact, it is very challenging for those affected. Most, if not all, need outside assistance to overcome this addiction. It is not as easy as just staying away from certain foods. The food addict's brain is waiting for those chemicals to be delivered so they may feel right with the world. Plus, remember we have food everywhere for all events. Our cultures are built around feasting on food. Imagine an alcoholic or heroin user running into large tables or counters of their addiction everywhere they went. In addition to get-togethers and family events, we have restaurants and stores that sell food everywhere. We can stay in our car and drive through picking up food from a window. In that sense, I see food addiction as one of the hardest to bring under control and maintain. Because you still need to eat food — always. If this is affecting you friend, I know there are new methods out there that people are having much success with.

Begin by contacting a food addiction specialist. There are many treatment options including online assistance, partial and full hospitalization. For group support options, begin with Food Addicts Anonymous and/or Overeaters Anonymous.

Holistic helpers include the flower essences of apricot, banana, American paw paw, and redwood.

Other Eating Disorders

Bulimia nervosa and anorexia cannot be classified as food addictions. However, since they involve food and many who have been sexually abused may suffer from these conditions, I wanted to mention them briefly. Experts have not identified what causes either of these ailments. They focus on a complex mixture of biological or genetic components combined with psychological and environmental factors.

With bulimia, the person suffering from this condition gorges on large quantities of food and then finds ways to quickly purge it from their system to avoid weight gain. This practice is dangerous as it often involves either vomiting, overuse of laxatives or enemas. There is another type of bulimic individual who will exercise excessively instead of purging. An individual with bulimia may feel very controlled by having to intake food and yet also battling the caloric consumption of it constantly. This can produce excessive anxiety, irritability and depression.

Anorexia involves the actual prohibition of food for one's self. In some instances, it can be a way the individual is enacting extreme control over something in their life. A distorted view of their bodies is common as they frequently believe they are overweight ... even when they are severely underweight. This can also be a dangerous, life threatening condition.

For both of these conditions, medication along with therapy is often necessary. Depending upon the individual's physical condition, hospitalization may be required for a time.

The flower essence American Paw Paw is recommended for anorexia specifically.

Nicotine

Unlike alcohol or mind altering drugs, an addiction to nicotine will not keep you from fully healing from sexual abuse. However, as you learn to value and love yourself on a deeper level, this is one addiction you will genuinely want to see go from your life because it can cause so many health problems to your body.

Nicotine is highly addictive. One therapist I had told me it was as hard to kick the nicotine habit as it is heroin. I believe her. While there are various methods of nicotine delivery, smoking is the most common. To a non-smoker, it is often inconceivable why people smoke. It stinks up everything. People are shunned from smoking in most public places. Yet, we have the same components going on with nicotine that we do with other addictions.

Nicotine works on the human body as both a sedative and stimulant. Indirectly, it releases dopamine tickling the brain's pleasure center. It increases levels of beta-endorphin. It lowers insulin by raising blood sugar and has an immediate effect on the adrenal glands that is stimulating in effect. There are many body functions affected by smoking including those in the gastrointestinal area, the heart, lungs, brain and hormones.

Bottom line of this addiction: Smoking is the most preventable cause of death. Yet, it may take considerable effort and determination on the part of those who want to beat this addiction. Additionally, it may take many tries with different methods. The American Heart Association also says nicotine from smoking is one of the hardest substances to quit. It is considered to be at least as hard as quitting heroin. Many people do beat their heroin addiction. Many people also beat their nicotine addiction.

Withdrawal from nicotine can produce many symptoms including:

- Irritability
- Attention Span Difficulties
- Focusing Issues
- Anxiety
- Emotional Overwhelm
- Cravings For The Substance

- ❖ Depression
- ❖ Moodiness

Continued nicotine use can lead to specific cancers that have been attributed to it. It affects the vascular system and heart with the intake of the substance immediately. Emphysema is often linked with smoking. The risk of stroke is greatly enhanced as well.

Methods to end nicotine addiction often include nicotine replacement therapies (NRT). These items vary in effectiveness for each individual. Nicotine replacement therapies can include patches, chewing gum, lozenges, inhalers and nasal sprays. Some people are able to use these products in moderation as they go through the withdrawal process.

Other NRT options include Bupropion which is technically an anti-depressant. It has helped some to withdrawal from nicotine. Some utilize the drug Varenicline (brand name Chantix). It is purported to work by blocking a receptor in the brain that is said to be activated by nicotine. While the person is taking it, they cannot get the same satisfaction and eventually quit their nicotine habit. Again, this works for some people, but not all. Both of these medications mentioned above do carry serious potential side effects for some. Other prescription drugs some are using to try and quit their habit include nortryptyline and clonidine. Both carry more serious potential side effects.

Having a support system in place to quit the nicotine habit can be very beneficial. Begin with nicotine-anonymous.org. Also ask clinics, physicians or nurses for resources in your area. To effectively beat the nicotine addiction, you need the right support, a well thought out plan, and determination.

Morning glory flower essence is recommended for symptoms from tobacco withdrawal. There are many other holistic helpers available.

While some individuals are vaping tobacco combined with other aromatic scents, they are still feeding the nicotine addiction. You can get custom blended vaping juices that do not contain nicotine and some do this to continue the actual smoking habit.

A new kid on the block is the Aromatherapy Diffuser Pen. Monq markets these products which they purport are inhaled through the mouth and exhaled through the nose. Only pure, clean essential oils are ingested that produce different effects for the user based on the scents.

Anytime you can use the essential oils of Lavender, Ylang ylang or Sweet Orange in your bath or other ways is beneficial. Plus, the more things smell so delicious, the more it makes you think about the stench of nicotine smoke. There are a number of ways to use essential oils. Put a few drops in an aromatherapy air diffuser and there are some made also for your vehicle that plug into the cigarette lighter. You can place a few drops in your favorite body lotion or hand cream. Remember when using essential oils you want to only use 3-4 drops as they are very potent and can cause skin irritation if too much is absorbed.

Some people wean off cigarettes by rolling their own cannabis. This will relieve stress, of course. However, some people crave cigarettes even more after smoking a joint. If marijuana is not legal in your area, you will want to avoid this option. Only consider this in regions where cannabis sativa is legal recreationally or medically.

Cardamom seeds are a spice that can be used by people kicking the tobacco habit. They have a strong, but tranquil aroma that helps relieve stress. Like aromatherapy, the scent and the sensation of chewing on the seeds is working as a temporary replacement for tobacco use.

If you can go without your nicotine, but just love smoking, you might want to consider some of the herbal cigarette blends on the market. The idea is to use the herbal cigs as a buffer while you are weaning yourself from the nicotine. Then, move forward with eliminating the smoking habit itself.

Hypnosis by a well qualified trained professional can help immensely as it works on removing the blocks and desire to smoke. While expensive and it may require more than one session, many have found success with this method of quitting.

Legal & Illegal Drugs

The use of illegal drugs is prevalent in all facets of societies throughout the world. One does not need to be a victim of any type of abuse to be a user of marijuana or cocaine. In fact, a study of over four hundred female adolescents indicated that just as many who had never been sexually abused partook in illicit drugs and alcohol. One notable difference, however, is that the females who had been sexually abused also often used stimulants, hallucinogens, tranquilizers or sedatives on a regular basis indicating some level of possible addiction (Harrison, et al., 1989).

Another factor that stood out is that most of the females used alcohol and other drugs at an earlier age than their counterparts who had not experienced sexual abuse. A definite difference was seen with the females who had experienced sexual abuse as they seemed to exhibit a need to self medicate.

A study conducted on male and female adult patients in treatment for drug abuse found that eighty-one percent of women had experienced sexual abuse which began at an average age of thirteen. Sixty-nine (69%) percent of the men reported sexual abuse beginning at an average age of eleven years old (Liebschutz, et al, 2002). Whether drugs used by these survivors are prescribed or not, the chance of them using the substances to numb their feelings is great.

There are more statistics that have been gathered that show similar results. Essentially, children who have been sexually abused are more apt to reach out and illegally use drugs. This attempt to alter their consciousness is understandable. They want to change how they are feeling or to avoid their feelings as much as possible. The problem is that this comes with high costs and dangerous risks that can impact them in numerous ways. This applies also to adult survivors.

Many illicit drug users may even begin within a social setting. When they see that they can feel "different" for a period of time while the drug is in their system, they want more of it. Before you know it, an addiction has formed. There is also usually experimentation with other drugs to see how they may affect the user.

While in the high state, mental conditions that have been plaguing the survivor may seem to disappear. They may feel confident, even if it is a temporary false sense of bravado. The illicit drug user may find themselves involved in crime to keep the whole thing flowing so they are constantly receiving the drugs they want to feel better.

Helpful Holistic Treatments

For all drug addictions, prescription or illegal, many modes of holistic therapy can be combined with regular conventional medical treatments to boost and increase success.

> ➢ Massage Therapy

- Nutritional Therapy
- Herbal Teas
- Homeopathic Preparations
- Aromatherapy
- Acupressure or Acupuncture
- Yoga
- Meditation
- Reiki or Energy Practitioner Work
- Flower essences of morning glory (opiates and nicotine), Self Heal or Skullcap

All of these can help with withdrawal symptoms and calming the emotions.

Other Addictions

Almost anything in the world can become an obsession which can lead to an addiction. I have known a couple of individuals who exercised so much it had truly become an addiction for them. Let's cover some common addictions.

Caffeine - If you need a lot of caffeine to go about your day, you may also have difficulties with good sleep. If we limit the amount of caffeine we have within a day, it will help us to fall into our natural biorhythms easily. Many experience headaches and other withdrawal symptoms when going with no caffeine at all. Unless abstaining entirely has been recommended by your physician, cutting your usage may be the best way to curb this if you feel it has become an addiction for you. Angelica is a flower essence often used for caffeine withdrawal, along with the flower extracts of live forever, lotus, nasturtium, nectarine, onion, Queen Anne's lace, redwood, coffee, sunflower, tuberose, Chinese wisteria and skullcap

Gambling - Studies have shown increased risk of pathological gambling addiction in sexual abuse survivors.

The flower essence of Four Leaf Clover can assist compulsive gamblers. Yes, seriously – four leaf clover!

Video Games - Anything that keeps you from normal interaction and responsibilities can be seen as addictive in nature, including the fun of playing these games. However, for some people, video games serve as a new habit to practice instead of the ones that kept them addicted to something more harmful.

Social Media - like video games, social media can be fun and help you interact even with others like you. It may be an outlet that keeps you from pursuing a dangerous addiction. As you use it, just keep in mind that it can also be addicting and the statistics do not show it always being something that is uplifting at all. In fact, it can have a depressing effect on many. A good rule of thumb for video games, social media, chat room sites, etc., would be to put a daily time limit on it.

Pornography - many people are addicted to viewing pornography. What they may not realize is they are supporting sexual exploitation and abuse by participating in it as a viewer. Behind the cameras, people are being hurt, taken advantage of and exploited. Porn has been called "the new drug". One of the most insightful internet sites you can check out is fightthenewdrug.org. They offer real facts with peer reviewed articles on how porn affects the brain, heart and ultimately, our world. A person afflicted with this addition may want to try the use of Pine Tree Sap to help with eliminating unhealthy thought patterns. Wood betony is a flower essence that balances sex drive with spiritual growth. This may also be useful.

Getting Help

There are many reasons to avoid getting help for an addiction. First, it means you are going to have to give up something that has become a big part of your life and way of living. It means change and that can feel monumental and difficult. Second, you may have shame surrounding the fact that you have this addiction. Third, you may not feel any methods you choose will work and give up before you have even started to try. You may fear judgment from professionals in addiction recovery fields. When you work with these ideas and drop the shame or embarrassment, you can begin to move forward. It takes work. Generally people need assistance to eliminate their addictions.

Utilizing holistic methods in addition to conventional ways can increase your success in battling addiction. Below is a sample war plan for ridding yourself of this monkey once and for all.

Make a Real War Plan

Depending upon your specific addiction(s), use the information below to come up with a plan that attacks this problem head on. Most people need a plan that is tailored just for them. By having a written plan you can post, follow and refer back to, you will experience more success. You may want to go over some of these ideas with any professionals or support persons you are conferring with as well. Remember also, within all wars you may lose a few battles. The point is to win the war. Be patient and forgiving with yourself. Forgive yourself for having an addiction. It is more common than you realize.

Determine what conventional methods will be part of your plan. This can include:

- Counseling
- Out-patient treatment
- In-patient treatment
- Prescription medications to ease withdrawal
- Group Therapy
- 12 Step Programs

- Mentoring Programs
- Replacement Therapies

Then, add holistic approaches which may include:

- Acupressure or Acupuncture
- Massage Therapy
- Reiki or Energy Work
- Yoga - Tai Chi
- Walking for Stress Relief
- Barefoot walking on grass or dirt (grounding)
- Hypnosis
- Chewing Cardamom Seeds
- Healthier Hard Candies
- Herbal Teas
- Flower Essences
- Healthy Snacks
- Affirmations
- Aromatherapy Inhaler or Infuser
- Meditation
- Chanting
- Prayer
- Tapping
- Reflexology
- Creative Visualization
- Journaling your feelings
- Coloring or Painting
- Singing and/or Dancing
- Animal or Equine Therapy

Two of the best overall flower essences to assist with withdrawal of addiction are morning glory and skullcap.

Realize that if you take the issue of addiction seriously enough to come up with a game plan, you have already increased your chances of winning. Even if you fall back into your addiction, pick up your war game plan again and keep going. Perhaps, you need to make some modifications to the plan. For instance, if you are trying to quit a particular substance and it is something that your friends or relatives do around you, the addiction is going to be harder to beat. You may have to pull away from some people while working on this.

I wish you much love and luck. Realize that even if you lose a battle or two, pick up your weapons you have chosen in this war and keep going. You will never win the war if you do not keep at this – readjusting your plan as needed along the way.

10 - Recognize Your Transgressor

Many times, you may believe it is only the one who perpetrated crimes against you that is the problem person in your life. During my journey, I have recognized that many people I was either related to or attracted into my life held personalities and traits that were a unique mixture of those who had abused me. When I saw this, it scared the hell out of me initially. I thought, "Wow, I am actually surrounded by the same energy I never wanted to be around." I knew I had to go deep inside myself once again, submerge myself into the sticky ugly mud to find out how and why this was occurring. This is often called visiting the shadow side of one's self. It is a place we generally want to avoid. I was no exception to this. Yet, I also wanted to be free of these very challenging, heart wrenching relationships I found myself in.

With a mixture of excitement and apprehension, I struggled for awhile to find a way to attack this problem. A part of me wanted to heal so badly and bust the negative patterns I saw within myself. Another part of me wanted to escape any way possible and ignore it. At times, my actions vacillated between these two modes. It seemed I would make two steps forward, one step back — two steps forward, one step back. The reason this was happening for me is the same as it is for anyone who is in need of trauma healing. I was running thought programs or patterns that needed to be recognized first, and then dealt with in a systematic way.

Perhaps you do not believe you have such programming patterns affecting your life. I hope you do not. It would make healing much swifter. Here are some signs that you may be still running a program from your subconscious that is not serving you. Begin by looking at your relationships and asking some questions.

Exploration of Relationships

This first question deserves considerable reflection without a quick answer. The complete answer may need to evolve over days or weeks. Question: After your experiences with those who hurt you, did you ever find yourself attracted to or involved with other people who shared traits of your abuser(s)?

Believe it or not, there can be a part of you that still attracts people who:

- Share strange little common mannerisms or traits of your abuser(s)
- Want to take instead of give
- Charm us initially, then show us the monster they are
- Dish out verbal, emotional, physical and/or sexual abuse

If you know that you are or have been engaged with someone sharing your abusers' traits, you need to really analyze the dynamics at play so you can avoid this in the future. How were you so attracted to them in the first place? Try to recall first contact with each person you have been in a relationship with, married to, etc. Perhaps it would be good to make a profile sheet on each of these people and I have provided a sample one that will prompt and assist you. You can download a pdf of it free at this link:: https://bit.ly/3jbcQIG

With this tool, you can print as many as you like to help you analyze and determine if friends and lovers in your life are falling into these patterns.

People who are toxic to us often have a mysterious air about them as if they are purposely making it difficult for you to know what makes them who they are in a complete way. This creates a curiosity within you and they know that. You may sense there is something that needs mending or fixed, especially as they recount how awful their last partner treated them or other injustices they proclaim. They may even believe everything they tell you or they may know they played a large part in destroying the relationship they had. Think about it, however, you really do not know how much damage they may have perpetuated upon the other person.

Often these individuals have an aloof air, making you work to be in their presence. You feel elated when they finally text, call or show up in person. This is part of creating the suspense and keeping you on unsure footing. It is a game played to hook you in. They are vague and non-committal, unless you have a lot of financial resources. If they discover that is the situation, you will be love bombed by them until they gain control over you and eventually drain you of those resources.

In any case, people like this are always attentive until they know they have you psychologically, physically or financially where they want you ... under their thumb. Unlike you, they have been studying you from the moment they saw or met you via chat. You mistake their questions as an interest in really knowing what you are about and that is not your fault. They take the information and use it against you in a variety of ways. They need to know what motivates you so they can find a way to offer up a self manufactured personality that fits your profile they have developed. In nature, this is the same way a predator studies their prey before pouncing on them.

In order to fully bloom and live the life you rightfully deserve, you must use both your intellect and intuitive sense to constantly be on the lookout for these individuals who have the capacity to destroy you.

Know your vulnerabilities

If you know that you have been attracting people into your life that do not treat you as you deserve, consider setting a rule for yourself to spend more time getting to know people prior to becoming so close. I know in love relationships this seems like it takes the fun out of it. We have movie and book inspired ideas about how we should fall so madly in love and everything will just work itself out. But holding onto that idea really keeps you in such a vulnerable position to be hurt and possibly abused again. People that end up abusing us do not do exactly what your original transgressor(s) did. Instead they do other things that, when analyzed, somehow produce the same result internally within you.

What can you do to prevent falling into a relationship with another abuser?

- In today's digital world, it's very easy to do actual background checks on people. There are companies available to do this for you for a really small price compared to your life and sanity.
- Look at all their activity online that you can find.
- Listen to what they say - are they a person who blames their last partner… or even the one before that?
- Go super slow - snail's pace. Don't allow them to rush you into this. Really get to know this person and observe their habits.
- Look at the friend/lover requirements further in this chapter and make your own as well.

Even though you are on a healing path, some of you may be engaged in a very dangerous situation where you are trauma bonded to at least one individual. If you are now or have found yourself in the past to be in a relationship that is unhealthy for you, trauma bonding can be a real cause. How can you know if this is going on? Here are some clues:

- Has anyone ever asked you why you stay in this relationship?
- Is the other person you are in the relationship with destructive to your emotions, physical self, your finances or property? In other words, do their words or actions hurt you and your position in life?
- Do you have feelings of just being stuck in this situation? However, when you break up with them, you find it so crazy and uncomfortable to be without them that you relent and bring them back into your life.
- You put more effort into their comfort than your own.
- You hold hope that they will change. In fact, they have told you they would and you know they are trying to do so – or at least they were.
- Disagreements and fights are too frequent.
- This person will abandon or hurt you when you do not behave the way they want you to.
- Other people in your life are worried about you and the effect this relationship is having on you. If the person you are trauma bonded with knows this, they will tell you things like, "they are just jealous; they want to break us up, etc."
- You just seem unable to end the relationship for good and maintain no contact with them.

> You stay because you are holding onto a promise they made you – the hope that they really will change.

Your friends or relatives cannot understand why you stay in this relationship. What they do not know is that trauma bonded relationships are quite complex on a psychological level. Often, we are repeating a pattern that occurred to us early on in life that involved the acceptance of abuse.

Many of these individuals very possibly suffer from narcissist or anti-social personality disorders. A few could be psychopaths which is extremely dangerous. Their tactics are always the same. They can be so charming when they want. After being kicked out or a fight, they will make promises they cannot keep. They may bring gifts to you or offer to take you certain places. This is all manipulation. It is known as love bombing. This is the period of time when they are exploding smoke bombs of love over your head to make you think there is something wrong with you and why in the world were you so upset with them to begin with. Yes, that's how it works. As the smoke above your head clears and you begin to question everything, they put forth their second line of defense. This involves making you think that what you believe is not real. And that is referred to also as gas lighting which is nothing more than invalidation, another subtle form of abuse. The toxic partner makes you think you are the crazy one, when it is really them.

It is very sad that these individuals suffer as they do. They will never have full beautiful relationships during their lifetime. At least that is my belief. Their brains are actually anatomically different than what we consider normal. We can surmise this from clinical brain mapping controlled tests. The first such test showed that those who had been diagnosed with narcissistic personality disorder contained less gray matter in the left anterior insula. This area of the brain is purportedly responsible for feeling emotional empathy. Subsequent mapping utilizing magnetic resonance imaging (MRI) also revealed less gray matter in the front paralimbic brain area. This portion of the brain is made up of the rostral and median cingulate cortex as well as dorsolateral and medial parts of the prefrontal cortex. Basically, this front portion of the brain where gray matter volume was less for those afflicted with NPD affects executive reasoning function (Schulze, et al, 2013).

Exploring how these gray matter deficits could affect another human, we can begin by looking at the specific functions identified as being controlled by these regions. The capacity for empathy jumps out first. Our ability to sense and feel what another may feel means we have compassion for others. The pre-frontal cortex area of the brain covers a larger area and is dedicated to a myriad of tasks. Executive functioning is one task of the brain's prefrontal cortex. This is our ability to make decisions; to set goals; to see ideas and tasks through to the end; develop patience or temperance instead of losing our temper.

Specific areas lacking in gray matter are the paralimbic regions. It is believed these deeper lying brain areas deal with our emotions and drives. The median cingulate cortex has been associated with formation of the emotions, memory and learning. Could this be why they promise to change and then forget?

The dorsolateral portion of the prefrontal cortex would be an area that helps people to self regulate — to make the appropriate choice in a situation. Example: Instead of robbing the bank with his two friends, John decided to bail and not be part of the situation, even though the money was needed and he was tempted. Those suffering from particular personality disorders may find it difficult to self-regulate impulses. I give you this anatomical detail in order to drive home the fact that these are people incapable of big change. They are wired differently.

One of my fears – just one – of leaving the toxic relationship I found myself in decades ago was that no one else would want me. In fact, my abusive partner had convinced me of that. Over time, he had repeatedly said things that made me feel like, "Damn, I better hang onto this, because it won't get any better." How wrong he was! How very wrong! Once I worked on healing by going to therapy and other tools, I began to see myself in a new light. I kicked him out of my place and began building a new foundation for myself. After some time, I met the person I have been married to now for twenty-five years.

Another fear I held is that if I did meet someone else, it would not be exciting like it was with my trauma bonded partner. But it was more exciting in a different way. You see, with the person you were bonded with through trauma, the excitement is the trauma itself – the back and forth dance you do; the arguments; and the makeup time periods.

In a healthy relationship, it is quite different. You share an intense closeness, sometimes so much that you are constantly reading each others' minds. You move in sync with one another, instead of against. And, your sex life takes on a better than ever dynamic because of the understanding and closeness you share.

Disagreements are infrequent as compared to the trauma bonded relationship. You are not trying to change this partner and they are not trying to change you. They love you in your perfectly imperfect state and you reciprocate those feelings. This gives you a great foundation to build from together as a team. In fact, you find that you both make a great team together.

The man I met when I had been on a healing path for a few years was sexier, more talented, kinder, and not afraid to be a family man as well. He held a maturity that was lacking in my trauma bonded partner. So don't sit and think you will never find anyone better. You can and you will, but first you must do the work.

If you find yourself in a relationship with someone who is toxic, make a plan to get out and stay out. Get well. Work on your healing. When I cut him out for good, I filled my time doing things that made me happy when I wasn't working. This included projects or places to go with my kids. It included a new hobby or two. It also included many late nights of reading every self-help book I could get my hands on, along with constantly plugging the small number of affirmations and related inspiration material that was available at the time into my brain. I kept going to therapy and when one method was not working, changed to another. I made it a huge priority to do whatever I needed to do to get well.

At the time, I was not doing it to meet someone else. I was doing it for me. This time period represented my first steps toward loving me and taking responsibility for all things in my life.

If you are in a toxic relationship that you know cannot be fixed, please consider making a plan to change up your life. Do not be afraid. I was afraid. But, I took the leap anyway. And it paid off in so many ways for me. I want the same for all survivors. I have faith in this process. I know it works.

Many times, especially with those abused during childhood, you had to learn to be very much on your own and to make the needs of others more important. You became very empathic to the feelings of those around you. You had to do this in a struggle for emotional, psychological or even physical survival. As an adult, you easily attract people who have toxic personalities. Some part of them recognized the part of you that would put up with their misbehaving ways. It did not seem like that at first. It seemed like love. But, it devolved into that easily with the personality dynamics going on.

If your life has been or is an emotional roller coaster, it is time to get off that ride and stop experiencing such extreme ups and downs. This would create stress for any human being.

All abuse survivors need a period of time alone - without toxic people around - to heal. Do not fear being alone because that state does not have to equate with loneliness. I happen to know that you can be in a relationship and still feel lonely. I bet many of you know that as well. During your alone time, you can actively work on your better life through therapy, reading, gaining knowledge about what has happened and how to correct things going forward. Otherwise, you will continually attract the same sorts of people who really may victimize you all over again - just in a different way. This can happen slowly or in a very swift manner. It is different in all circumstances. But, the thing that is always the same is that you have the potential to break free from this cycle.

That is all it is - a pattern that is repeating. Once you realize this is the mode you have been operating within - and often it is with the eyes and ears of another that brings you to that sweet conclusion - you have the power to change it. Unfortunately, you will never change those toxic people in your life. Forget about that. It will not happen. Most of them promise to change - heard that many times myself in the past. They will not. They might change for a week and then they are back to the way they always were. As you change, the things around you will change. This is the power of taking charge of your life and journey of healing.

Mirror, Mirror

Some of you are being re-victimized now. Perhaps, you know this or maybe you do not recognize it. What do I mean by that? You have possibly found yourself in a relationship with people who mirror the treatment you received during your abuse on some level. Let's look at some possibilities that could happen for an abuse survivor.

Relationships really can mirror where we are at mentally within ourselves. When I first learned that many years ago within spiritual teachings, I really had a hard time embracing this. It took awhile. Basically, what we experience in a relationship with someone is that they are mirroring something we need to look at within us. And I remember thinking, yes but I am not like the other person. I'm not cruel like them. And of course, you are probably not. What you are is a person that needs to work on figuring out why you would allow someone like that in your life.

The metaphorical idea of the mirror is a very useful tool. Sometimes, we can determine where we are in our recovery by examining the quality of the relationships we have around us. If we are married or partnered with someone who displays behaviors we know are damaging to us, it is certain that we have healing to do. For some survivors, this can be a hard thing to accept. Many times, they want to blame the other party. We might say, "It's their problem" They have narcissistic or anti-social personality disorder. This could be true. However, this puts you, the survivor, in a weak position. When we blame and do not look at our own participation in relationships, we are not in a position to take back our power.

If you are in a relationship with someone who is not good for you, you must ask yourself why. Is it for financial reasons? Can you make it on your own without them?

Most instances I have seen, these people are draining you – emotionally, physically and financially. You are a supply source for them. Once you are finally an empty well, they move on to another supply source. Many times, these individuals will already have another one lined up.

Persons who fall under the umbrella of narcs (narcissistic personality disorder) or sociopaths can be very charming and cunning. They manipulate you into thinking that you are the problem – not them. If you would just do as they want and fall in line, everything would work out. Yet, it doesn't. There are at least two outcomes that occur from you acquiescing and doing as the toxic personality requests.

First, your own spirit within will be crying out at times, "not fair – not right". Second, you will suffer emotionally to a very large degree. This will result in anger that is stuffed down inside, soon turning into depression. The only lift you get is perhaps after a fight with this person and the love bombing that occurs afterward in the make up phase.

Dr. Wayne Dyer once said, "When you don't make peace with your past, it will keep showing up in your present."

It also helps to become familiar with words and actions that people with personality disorders utilize. Knowledge is power and knowing the signs is critical to keep you from being victimized again. When you can react out of logic and true knowledge, rather than pure emotion or fears, it helps. When it comes to phrases that your significant other may throw at you frequently, here are the most common:

They tell you that you are crazy. Usually, this is a form of gas lighting where they attempt to make you believe that what happened did not really happen. It is a form of invalidation. Although subtle, gas lighting is a form of abuse.

They say you are overly sensitive, instead of justifiably bothered by something. Here is one example of how that may play out. Your love interest tells you they will call you on Friday afternoon about plans for the weekend. They never call or text. Saturday morning and you still have not heard from them. Saturday around 1pm, you finally hear from them.

When you ask why they did not call, they make excuses. Perhaps your love interest states that they worked late and so tired they just fell into bed. Or, perhaps your love interest tells you they went out with the guys or girls and had a little too much to drink and just forgot.

When you let them know you don't like being forgotten or treated like that, they say you are being overly sensitive. Are you?

I don't think so. If someone tells me they will call on Friday about our plans for the weekend and they don't, I may worry about their welfare. Even if they worked late or went out on the town with friends, they could call or text and say something.

They say you are stupid – for any reason. People that love you don't say things like that. It's not acceptable.

They indicate by their treatment of you that you are not good enough, don't measure up or are just worthless. Love never does that!

When they fear you splitting with them or they want to get back into the relationship with you they may say, "No one will ever love you like I do." Really, how does this person love you? Does love behave the way they do?

They tell you, "No one will want you now". Never believe this --- never! It's just not true.

Perhaps maybe not the exact words are used, but are the feelings the other person is putting on you similar as the abusers in your life? Think about that. If you are in a relationship (or were) and you step back and listen to the two of you interacting, what is being communicated in the way of feelings?

It is very likely that a scenario is playing out that is much like the way your abuser made you feel. Spend some time thinking and analyzing this very closely.

There are so many examples of people – both men and women who find themselves in relationships that are nothing more than a strange mirror of the abuse they endured earlier in life. How is it that they attract this? It all comes down to where you are resonating and what you will accept or go along with.

Many survivors have an intuitive, empathic nature. Those with particular personality disorders are consciously and unconsciously looking for those attributes in a partner. They want to find someone who is very kind, supportive and who "understands" their situation or problems.

You will find your emotions going up and down in this kind of relationship. As soon as they feel they may have pushed you to the edge of no return, they flip and change. At this point, they may do things that seem like acts of love or adoration. It is important to remember that love is something they can only feel for themselves and even then, not a true love of self worth. They need people like you to make them worthy. To support them and tell them yes, the whole world is bad because they don't see how great you are.

Here are some hypothetical situations that are very common in these types of relationships.

John and his partner have been living together for over a year. He has a steady job and is paying most of the living expenses for the couple. John is a sexual abuse survivor. His partner goes through jobs frequently and constantly needs loans or help with certain things. The partner is loving and the relationship feels very alive and exciting during those times when the partner wants something. A good portion of the time, however, the partner is out of touch and downright nasty and negative to be around. John feels like he is perhaps not good enough at times because his partner tells him little things that are specific criticisms. If John accidently misses answering a phone call from his partner because he was in a meeting at work, all hell breaks loose with accusations and cussing. John cannot tell if this control he feels from his partner means he is really loved or just being manipulated. His partner does not want him to see his other friends from work or even his parents, saying negative things about each.

When John finally puts his foot down and threatens to kick his partner out, suddenly the mood changes and there are promises that the partner will change and not act like that again. Two weeks later, the same behavior continues.

Let's dissect this. John was traumatized and abused by an adult when he was a young teen. In addition to having to meet the demands sexually of this adult, he also had to make his whereabouts and activities known constantly. This went on for a long enough period of time that it is possible John sees this as normal relationship dynamics on some level without being conscious of it. The logical part of John knows the behavior he is experiencing in his current relationship is not right or fair. Yet, his emotional expectations are set into his neural pathways about what a relationship consists of. He is conflicted as this tells him otherwise.

It will take John overriding this emotional expectation. In order to do this, he will need to value and love himself first. He must be willing to let this relationship go also, even if it hurts. He must develop a hard line when it comes to ignoring the false promises his partner will make to stay in the relationship. It will be tough because his personality disordered partner will really come on strong now with promises, love bombing and finally anger and threats when John does not relent. There may be stalking. John might have to involve the police. It could get messy, but it will be necessary for John to move from this relationship that is going nowhere to healing and eventually having one that is a match to his healed survivor self.

Another scenario:

Marla is a sexual abuse survivor whose traumatic events began early in life at the hands of her older brother. The brother threatened Marla with public embarrassment and told her she would upset the entire family. He also told her he would do the same to her younger sister if she told. Marla endured her brother's abuse out of fear and shame. She left home as soon as she could, running away at fifteen where she encountered more abusers as she tried to survive on her own. This set up a pattern in her life.

Things were beginning to look up for Marla. She found a decent job at a nice restaurant where she could make enough tips to afford to be on her own or stay with her current roommate easily. Then she met Billy. He was hot and had charisma coming out every pore of his being. Billy had money too. From speaking with the other servers at the restaurant, Marla knew it came from illegal endeavors like drugs and weapons. But Billy's persona had captured her. What did Billy see in Marla? She was young for sure but legal at eighteen now. More than that, Marla was pliable. Billy knew he could mold her into what he wanted and felt he needed.

Like so many relationships, it started out hot and the love bombing was going on constantly. Marla felt Billy was her one true love. Billy knew Marla was a thing – a relationship. Love? What's that all about anyway, he thought?

Billy seemed like a protective big brother in a way. He moved Marla into his incredible house and gave her the use of one of his expensive vehicles. Soon, however, he began to be very controlling and verbally abusing Marla. He would tell her that she better not eat something when they went out to dinner because he could not put up with her gaining even a couple of pounds. Marla had left the education system early in life and Billy used that against her calling her stupid often. Soon, he wanted Marla to participate in things sexually that she did not feel comfortable with including group sex. He taunted Marla and tried to make her feel jealous as he had sex right in front of her with another female. The only reason this hurt Marla is because it activated fear inside of her. If Billy tossed her aside for another female, where would she be then? She would lose the nice house and car, the expensive things he lavished upon her.

On one occasion to test Billy's feelings for her, she had sex with two men at once during a party ... right in front of Billy who attempted to not look fazed by this. Later, after much drinking and partaking of drugs, Billy went crazy on Marla verbally and beat her badly. For months after that, things were not the same. He was distant, mean and withholding in all ways. Eventually, Marla called her old roommate and begged for help to get away from him.

Do you see what Marla is setting up in her mind? If I do what Billy wants and give him what he asks for, I will be okay. This is almost exactly the dynamic that went on with her brother as a child. If I do what he wants, everyone else in the house will be okay.

It's really all about unconsciously mimicking the trauma bonding you endured before. You are recreating a set of conditions that result in particular feelings of familiarity. That is what **you** feel you cannot let go of – not the other person. They are just a mirror of what is going on with you and what you need to change.

Breaking up with these people is difficult – very hard to do! You are likely to go through as many emotions during and after the break up as you did staying in the relationship. However, the difference is this time, if you stay no contact and heal, your life will begin to change.

Who you attract will change. But it takes work and time. You will have to be tough with yourself because now you will interpret your aloneness to be loneliness. You will have to sit and look at you and what your needs are. Now, you are not going to be living your existence for what the narc or sociopath needs, but what you desire in life. You will discover your deepest insecurities, but you will heal from this knowledge and taking steps to alleviate it for good. It takes loving yourself enough to say no more abuse. No more crap from other people. I care about me and if you don't hit the road and don't come back. You will become stronger than you've ever been and, as you heal more, have a chance to find your true purpose.

Continuing a relationship with a toxic personality person can alter your entire life. I have seen it take people's lives because they did not get away from the abuse.

It is an act of loving yourself to be selective when you choose to partner with someone. It shows you are willing to be alone rather than fall for the next bad relationship. You have the power. What is the power? It is powerful to step up for yourself – to be your own champion and know that you will speak up and say yes or no to situations that come along.

What if you slip up? It's okay. We all do. This is a journey through the cocoon and it takes some time to emerge as a butterfly. When you know you're slipping, reach out and ask for help from others who can be supportive of what you are going through. Devise a way back out of what you have gotten yourself into.

Do you really want to have better control over your life? Do you want to live a life that is more like a good dream than a bad one? If so, you must really commit to your healing. It will mean making some hard decisions at times. It will mean looking at dark sides of yourself that you may not want to. I can tell you that the reward is great if you are willing.

It is possible that, along the way, you have picked up patterns playing out in real time constantly. Sometimes you can see these patterns and other times not.

Healing is something you engage in day by day as you travel this journey. You come to high hilltops within that walk when you are looking down on how much you have traveled, feeling elated at how far you have come. But you still may not have arrived – okay? It seems there are always more deep valleys to traverse. This is very individualized to each person and their abuse that occurred. It involves many things. There are therapies available that can and perhaps should be explored. These will help lay down new neural pathways assisting you in feeling and acting differently. However, without opening up your feelings and looking at the ugly stuff, the wound cannot begin to heal.

You also need kind, helpful and knowledgeable guides along the way with your journey. This would include very good friends you can count on, self help materials like this and most of all, qualified professionals who can assist you.

Often, we can look at who we are in relationship with and see mirrored back to us what we need to do to heal. When we see that reflection and have the courage to do so, life changes for us. It's difficult. I know how hard it is. But remember, there are many willing to help you make the steps toward a better future where you are healed, find your larger purpose and finally have the better relationship that you deserve.

Why would you bloom in a garden full of weedy characters? This is what we need to ask ourselves. Why do I not care enough about myself that I would be with this person? Why am I having trouble feeling I deserve more? What lies at the root of that? Always, it is our wounds that we carry deep inside. They make us feel that we are not enough; that we are not worthy of better love. And I am not excusing any of the behavior of unsavory individuals. Instead, I am saying that you have lost your power when you are blaming the other person. You stand in your power when you look at what the other person is doing and you look at yourself and say, "Why would I be around this?" One way or another, you have the power to move from that relationship to no relationship. It can be super beneficial and speed your healing to be without a relationship for awhile. Almost always without exception, if we move from one relationship where we think that person is the problem into another without the time period of healing and figuring out what is going on within ourselves, we find ourselves in another relationship that mirrors the one we were in before. It is the same play with different actors but about the same outcome and story line.

When it comes to relationships, it is a learning curve because you are unconsciously attracting and hooking up with people that often mimic your abuser in some way. As you realize this and correct it, you change internally. You learn to recognize these things easier and faster and stay away from them … no matter the attraction you have or level of loneliness you may feel. If you have filled your life with other activities that bring you a creative emotional outlet or improve your skill set in life, you will not feel such a pull toward those who are not in your best interest.

When we put people together and their energies do not match up, we feel resistance. When this occurs, one option is to avoid those people in our life, especially if they ignore preferences or push boundaries. At times, we must be around others that rub us the wrong way. It could be at a job where a co-worker is a huge problem for you. One option is to build an invisible wall around you that is like an iridescent light bubble. Use your imagination to do this. Everything you do not want to let in bounces off this protective bubble.

Anatomy of Relationships

By instituting requirements on who will be your friend or lover, you show respect and love for yourself. Relationships require ground rules that everyone is aware of to flourish and be the best they can be. Likewise, you need to avoid abuse or even plain old drama to bloom to your potential.

It can be very challenging to attract and maintain good relationships post abuse. The word "good" is somewhat subjective. What one person believes is good, another may not. Let us explore some definitions of what it can mean in relationships with others.

Friendships

You have people in your life that you know and converse with that could be just acquaintances. This could include neighbors, co-workers and friends of others. Then, you have people you consider a friend – sometimes a very good friend. What are the major differences between acquaintances and good friends?

Generally, you would have lower expectations of an acquaintance. You would be more hesitant to share certain things with them because you have not developed a trust level with that person. When it comes to friends, we really need to be able to trust them. A good friend will be willing to listen to you, allowing you to vent. Likewise, you as their good friend reciprocate by allowing them to talk to you about their concerns or situations.

A good friend should be able to keep a secret. If you cannot trust them to do so, it affects the level of the friendship, really taking it down to the acquaintance level. You would not confide or share secrets with an acquaintance.

Good friends typically share similar values such as personal integrity and honesty levels. For instance, you and your friend may think little white lies are okay and even sometimes necessary to carry out with others. However, you would both be honest with each other. Or, you may both believe the truth should always be spoken. Whatever the stance is, you will both generally share about the same feelings and opinions on this because if you didn't, challenging moments could occur to affect the friendship.

At times, a good friend might accidentally say or not do something that hurts your feelings. However, it is unintentional and could just be the way you interpreted a situation. A major difference is that a good friend will never intentionally hurt, belittle or abuse you in any way. Good friends treat each other with respect.

Yet, should you end a valued friendship over one mishap or secret revealed? I think it is important to realize we all make human mistakes. A conversation should be had between the two of you to confront the situation and allow things to hopefully go forward again. Like many things, this has to be determined on a case by case basis.

Lovers - Partners – Spouses

It is very likely that everything you required for a good friend, you also require for a romantic partner. You could include all or most of those items and have additional requirements. Generally, in order to be a romantic partner or spouse, they need to be faithful sexually. Although I am aware there are some relationships where there is a mutual decision to have open sexuality with others. A word of caution here is that you are not being manipulated by your partner into believing this is a good thing if you don't really feel that way at a core level. A good test question for this is: if you suddenly decided you wanted to not be in an open sexual relationship, would your partner respect your decision and cease the extracurricular activities?

A love partner or spouse should ideally be able to tell you if something is not working for them and you should feel comfortable relating that as well. This goes back to the honesty and transparency present in a good friend. In order to have a long lasting love relationship, we must be good friends first. It cannot be all about physical attraction and those types of exchanges. That won't last. Sex is a flimsy foundation to build upon in a relationship.

You must be able to communicate with each other without fear of the other one being angry or abandoning you. If that person cares for and loves you, they will listen when you are feeling dissatisfaction of some sort. Just remember that you do have to learn or know skills to talk to your partner in this manner. If you are blaming and accusatory, anyone's first reaction will be to defend their position. This often leads to arguments in even the best relationships that are not toxic. A great way to tell your partner what you feel dissatisfaction with is to simply state how you feel. Here is an example.

Your partner has taken to working overtime and is gone so much that when you do see them, they are too fatigued to help you with something you need or plan time together. You can say something like, "right now I feel that I cannot get the help I need because you are away so much." This is much better than saying, "Because you are working overtime, you are not here to help me."

Or, you could say, "I really miss having our special time together while you are working so much. Is there anything we can do to remedy that?" A statement like this opens up a dialogue between the two of you. If you say, "our relationship is suffering because you work so much." This has a totally different effect on your partner.

I am not suggesting that you coddle your partner or have trepidation or fear about bringing up things that need to be spoken about or resolved. All I am saying is to think about how you say things before you speak. Is there a way that you can say the same thing without the other person feeling attacked? Wouldn't you do that with a friend?

Here are some important things you want in your love relationship or marriage. You want a partner who is financially responsible. This does not mean they need a perfect credit score, but it does mean that they make real attempts to settle debts, save some money if possible and be responsible about their money and spending choices.

Why is this important? Financial issues are one of the main reasons people begin to experience stress in relationships. Let's face it. It can mean the difference between you having a place to live or not. There are also situations where the financial burden is placed upon one person in the relationship solely. Hopefully, this load is not upon you. This is tremendously unfair if the other person is capable of making money.

You also want a love partner that is emotionally available to you. In return, you are emotionally available to them. You each care about the feelings of the other.

Your love partner should have boundaries that you find acceptable and are in alignment with your core beliefs. They should also respect and accept your boundaries.

I think sometimes as survivors we might believe that we won't find the right kind of person for us. I am a firm believer there is someone out there for you to partner with that is healthy mentally. You will find that person more attractive, loving and kind than the one you have been hooking up with. It's so important to realize this and have a little faith and trust in the universe. It's that negative ninny part of you that is saying you are not good enough; don't deserve; won't match up; or whatever words it may say in your brain. Tell it you hear it, but it is wrong and let's get some affirmations going that attract healthy relationships to you.

At one point in my life, I had a long term off and on relationship with a character afflicted with anti-social personality disorder. I didn't know that he had it. But, I found out because this guy was an additional catalyst for me to seek counseling. Why did I keep letting him come back into my life? Why was I so weak about this instead of strong? All of my friends knew he was no good for me and tried to tell me often. Jeez, they were patient with me and still remained my friends. I'm sure they could not figure it out. I had trouble seeing it also -- until one day during therapy. It was on that day that I realized his personality was a strange combination of my two main abusers in life.

And that brings us back to your beginnings – your early life and the one you may have now with family. Our family of origin relationships can be some of the most daunting to overcome in life. Our families or the people who cared for us growing up were like pulling the wild card out of a huge deck. Sometimes we got lucky. Often, we did not. Our family of origin, or the lack of family, can bring up so many issues for us. We may be close to one or two persons within our families and have trouble getting along with many others. Or, we may enjoy the company of almost all of our family, but then there is that one person who cannot be trusted. This is very common. Most abuse survivors have experienced situations within family units that are extremely distressing.

The profound effect this has upon us often cannot be measured. We also walk around in our life from early adulthood on often unknowingly choosing relationships in our lives that mirror the dynamics that went on as children. This is just another reason that the inner child work is critically important to do.

Some of you came from a family where the problems have been so intense you no longer see those relatives.

There is nothing wrong with that. Some survivors may have experienced abuse within the family unit and still connect with some of their family. Unfortunately, we cannot change our family. But, we can regulate how much they are active or not in our life. Due to the fact that certain family members can evoke such intense feelings from us, it could be a situation where distance is needed. If there is a true toxic situation, your boundaries might even include no contact with certain members on a temporary or permanent basis.

There are so many different types of trauma we can endure during life. This one – the trauma of being in a relationship with a toxic personality – is self inflicted. Understand that fully. You are going to have things happen in life that you don't have control over … just like the sexual abuse trauma you endured. If we knowingly or unknowingly hook up with people who are toxic and retraumatize us, this is a choice now at this point. I realize for many it may not be a conscious choice. But the moment you know, you have the power to make changes and take control of your current life and future.

Know that as long as you stay in a toxic, trauma bonded relationship, you will be a victim. Even if you are a survivor in the sense that you survived your abuse of the past, you have now slipped back into the role of victim. And that is not a pretty place to be. It is not a powerful place to be. Where you need to take yourself as a sexual abuse survivor is into a position of thriving. It takes time. You can do it. First, however, you must see the things that are tripping you up in life so that you can get to the good stuff.

11 – Preferences

By giving relationships structure and stating expectations, you bypass many problems. First, you increase your chances of not hooking up with the wrong individuals. They won't like your rules. Second, when the rules are known, it is much easier to play. You cannot sit down and play a board game without stating the rules up front — although I have seen situations like this. All of a sudden, one of the players does something and another player calls them out. But, they did not know the rules until now.

As a survivor, you need to have a clear voice coupled with firm confidence to create healthy boundaries in all areas of your life. From the workplace to the home, boundaries are easily ignored by others. Let's work on fixing that for the beautiful future you want to create.

The word "boundaries" is used so much in the healing field that some of us just want to throw up when we hear it. A survivor may think, "Yeah, yeah, I know. It's my fault because I don't have good boundaries." We are going to take a different approach to this.

First, let's use the word preferences. I want you to become comfortable stating your preferences to all people in your life - your boss, children, partner, parents, everyone! Part of being truly healed is your new found ability to not allow people to take advantage of you. It is a critical, important skill that you build. As you state your preferences to others with more ease, your entire world around you begins to change.

At first, the changes you make in stating your preferences may seem harsh. This could feel like a very radical change to the personality you have been displaying to other people prior to now. It is likely you will receive backlash from those around you that do not want to see changes come about. This is normal and expected until they see over time you are serious about not only stating your position, but being a champion for it. Having preferences and enacting them does not mean you are completely inflexible. Instead, you have firm ideas of what is acceptable to you and what is not. You stand by those principles and support them with not just words, but action if you must.

For some of you, this learning of preferences and how to enforce them is critical to keep you from being sexually abused again. Statistics show a significant percentage of child and adolescent sexual abuse survivors are victimized again as adults. Often, this occurs because the survivor still has so much to work through. At the base of their feelings, we usually find shame and/or self loathing. It is so important to work through those issues and engage in activities that can help build confidence and self-worth.

Let me be very clear that being sexually abused is never your fault. No blame lies with you — but with the perpetrator. For further clarification, if we are operating in a lower personality mode and have not healed sufficiently, it can be easier to fall into the hands of someone who wants to hurt us.

Survivors often feel they are quote "ruined". At times they believe no one would want them in their life – no one will ever want to be with them. This is not true. This is a false preconception.

If you hold that type of feeling or belief it is because you do not value and love yourself enough. It's really all about you – not other people. When you love yourself and value your existence – this gift of life you have been given, your world really changes. You will see that who you attract changes. Working on enacting your preferences is an act of love for yourself. Yes, you have some work ahead to heal, but it is so worth it. Your tasks will be to work through the shame portion first and also address any addictions you have that can interfere with healing such as alcohol or drug abuse. Another sad fact is that many child sexual abuse survivors are sexually abused again later while they are intoxicated or high. Their guard is down and an opportunistic predator comes along, taking advantage of that fact. Again, this is not their fault for the crime occurring. Rather, it is just another predatory type individual taking advantage of a situation.

For those who have accomplished considerable healing, you may experience a different type of abuse in the form of toxic relationships. I spoke about the dynamics going on in these types of relationships and how trauma bonding is usually involved in the previous section. Some survivors fall into toxic relationships because they are unknowingly attracting this, entering into relationships with those that match previous abusers on some level. Once this pattern is recognized, you can remedy it. Most of the time, it will mean ending that relationship and working more on your healing so you attract people around you that are not toxic and abusive. This is true for family, work and friend relationships as well.

People will treat you well or not so well based upon what they sense you will tolerate. Clearly stating your preferences and speaking up for yourself – being that champion for your inner child keeps things in check so you are not continuing to be hurt on any level.

Many times, the survivor is not stating their preferences in a real clear manner. If they were, the relationship probably would not have happened. The toxic individual would have gone on to an easier "victim". Yes, victim. Because when we do not take up for ourselves and have our own set of rules of engagement, we are very likely to slip into the victim role. The mostly healed individual still needs to work on self love in a major way.

When they do this, they will not allow people to treat them in a manner that is not loving. It's just that simple.

In the past, we were forced to give up some of our power to others who victimized us. Unconsciously, we keep doing this in unique, different ways long after the sexual abuse has ended. Many times we are not aware it is happening. Operating from a feeling of not feeling good enough, we fear people will pull away, punish us in some way, or abandon us if we state our rules of engagement.

This can mean that we allow not only our partners to walk all over us, but any children we have as well. It can mean that we stay working in an environment that is extremely unhealthy for us.

I will say it again – if we really love ourselves, we will not allow this to be the life we are living.

What is keeping us from feeling this love and respect that we must have for us?

Fear – all of it is just fear often combined with negative self-talk.

What do we fear?

- Change
- Abandonment
- Confrontation – we all want to avoid the wrath of another.

Change

You do not have to be an abuse survivor to have fears surrounding change in your life. Almost everyone feels discomfort making changes, whether it is slight or massive in nature. Change is hard. It requires that we make choices. Once a choice is made, it is followed by a firm decision. Decisions sometimes require discipline or follow-through. None of this sounds fun, but it is all how we look at it.

First, change is constantly happening in our world – actually in the entire universe. Change is flow and things are always moving into different positions creating new outcomes. This is a natural principle we can see all around us. The seasons change along with the movement of our planet and constellations in space. Our moon moves every twenty-eight days from dark to full and bright. Its pull affects changes in the tide of the oceans and even the behavior of earth's inhabitants.

Your skin on your body right now will be different in cellular structure in thirty days. If you are older like me, your gray will make another appearance soon because you are changing physically from infancy on. Change is all around us. You are here because you desire change on some level. Think about it. Many times we want circumstances around us to change for the better. Yet, we secretly self-sabotage our efforts to enact change out of fear. Change is different. To make it happen, you must make firm commitments and actually do things to see the change happen.

Occasionally, you have moments where change is instant. This can especially be true with mindsets we carry. More often, change is gradual as you work upon your healing. This is just one more reason I stress reciting affirmations out loud or in your mind on a very regular basis. Affirmations help to create change inside of you. Change inside begins to reveal changes on the outside.

Now, let's look at the fear of abandonment. This is pretty self explanatory. What happens just prior to being abandoned in some way? Rejection occurs. Don't we all fear rejection? If I were a surgeon ready to fix your problem and could remove the fear of rejection from you, this would solve so many problems. How can you remove the fear of rejection? Stop giving a hoot about what others think. This is difficult because we all want to be liked. Yet, when you begin stating your preferences, some are going to pull the old, "Well If you won't see it my way, I don't want anything to do with you." So be it.

Some people will finally respect you for stating your preferences. Most will not because they are just as timid about change as you might be.

Many of us worry about not being perceived as nice. This must not be the driving concern. Being too compliant and nice can get you into situations where you are being taken advantage of. It is time to not worry about being nice, but being respected.

Soon, you learn that you can be a nice person who is respected because you state your preferences in a thoughtful way that does not threaten others. In the beginning, you may need to be stern with the people in your life. You may not sound nice. But these are the people who have been walking on top of you for awhile. It will take some shocking statements from you for them to begin to see that you are changing and you are no longer going to tolerate the treatment you are receiving. Dropping the need to be liked by everyone is a major accomplishment in your healing journey.

Confrontation is feared while we assert our preferences to those we have been in relationships with for awhile. Whether it is a parent, child, co-worker, or romantic partner, we fear getting into a verbal fight. For some, verbal confrontations lead to physical ones. If this is the case, you really must consider getting out of that relationship permanently. If the prospect of physical abuse exists, the fear of being physically hurt will be large enough to keep you from stating your preferences. In this type of situation, end that relationship as soon as you possibly can before you begin stating preferences or putting limits in place. I know this is much harder to do than I have made it sound here. It can be very difficult with many different components interfering in ending the relationship. Get help from others you can trust. You may really need this assistance, even if it is just moral support.

You must end physically abusive relationships ... or one where that potential is a sure outcome if you state your preferences. You will never be able to break free from your past and heal if you do not do this

Limits

Another way I would like to look at boundaries is limits. Boundaries are not just preferences you have but also limitations. If people know what our limit is, they will react one of two ways. They will respect that limit or boundary, or they will try to push against it. This tells you much about the other person.

Many of you listening have children or know others with kiddos. All children from toddler age on will test the limits and try to break some rules here and there. They are pushing against the boundaries to see how far they can go. This is natural and normal. Children will continue doing this through adolescence and many do beyond that stage as well. When adults are continuing to engage in it, they are attempting to take advantage of another. It is not really a kind practice. If you respect other people, you don't push their limits.

Finally, it is important to understand that you are not making rules for others – not at all. When you let others know your limits or preferences, you are simply allowing them to know what is okay with you and what is not. How they treat that information is their response. If they do not respect it, you must be willing to take action.

Being able to let others know our preferences – what we will allow and what we will not – is critical to creating a beautiful life that contains less drama and strife. However, as you change and allow others around you to know your limits, you may initially experience tough moments.

For the most part, you are going to need to be tough with yourself. You must be willing to act when people are not respecting these preferences you have put forth. If you tell a teenage child of yours that you will no longer tolerate them leaving their dishes for you to wash for them, you must be willing to put some sort of consequence in place if they break the rule. For instance, you might tell your teen that they will lose certain privileges they now have if they leave the dirty dishes. Instead of washing the dishes for them, you might put them all in a box or plastic bin and allow them to collect. Let them know you will consider reinstating the privilege when they have washed and put away those dishes.

With adults in your life, you are not always in a position to take away specific things from them. However, you can take other actions. But, you must really be willing to act and follow through to show this person what your limit is.

For instance, let's say that your partner is quite negative and says things that are hurtful to you – words that are mean and really serve no purpose other than to put you down. Here are two possible outcomes:

Before you put your preferences forth and let this person know your limits, you may have responded with anger, tears, silence or words like: "You can't talk to me like that." This is not effective enough.

Now that you are putting preferences in place, an effective statement and action would be:

"I do not allow people to talk to me that way, including you. That is purely abusive and it is not part of what I want to be around any longer."

The action: At this point, depending upon the circumstances, you need to part ways at least temporarily with this person. You could pick up your keys and go for a drive, leaving without saying where you are going and letting them know you will not be around such behavior. If this person is living off you primarily at your house, you can demand they leave until they speak kindly to you. Either way, there must be some sort of actual consequence to allow this person to know they have hit a wall with you – yes, your boundary. There is a limit now in place.

This is a mild example. I know some of you are embroiled in relationships with people that are much more abusive and toxic. Each circumstance is different. If you fear for your physical welfare and safety, do not enact preferences, but seek a way to get out of that relationship for good. Because putting preferences in place where you had none before can bring out the worst behavior in others. So, it is important to first be safe. Once you have another relationship in the future, you must allow that person to know from the first introduction onward that you have limits and preferences. You need to let them know from the very first how you expect to be treated.

Some key points to remember in this journey regarding your preferences and what you will allow in your life are:

Self Love

The simple act of caring for one's self helps build self worth that may be lacking due to abuse. Negative patterns and self-talk can be interfering with your recovery on a constant basis. By making self care a priority, this is a holistic way to improve self esteem and self love.

Loving yourself does not mean you cannot love others. It means that you will be more fully open to love others in a deep, meaningful, but fair way. You will allow others to fix their problems instead of you feeling as if you need to rescue them. Self love means you stop ignoring the inner thoughts and signals your soul cries out for and begin to listen first — then take action to fulfill them. In a very real way, just the fact that you are listening to these words is an act of self love. It indicates you are receptive to changes you know on some level would be very beneficial for you. Throughout this book, just about everything you are absorbing and doing as exercises or new life habits is an act of self love.

It is extremely important to work on this continually. Look at ways you may not be making yourself a priority. Do you take care of the needs of other adults around you, rather than your own? Do you make their feelings, moods, or preferences more important than the ones important to you? If so, these are areas to work on to develop more self love.

Safety

It would be nearly impossible to heal if you do not feel physically safe. When we are in an abusive environment, it can be difficult to set limits or initiate preferences with someone who will hurt us. The abusive relationship is the first thing to address in your life. How can you get out of it as gracefully as possible? Seek help and advice for this from qualified sources and perhaps close friends and/or family.

Only set limits with those you know will not hurt you physically. You may be emotionally hurt because of the need to break up the relationship. You may experience temporary financial turmoil due to a split. Yet, you must do this to heal. There is no exception. Once this toxic person is out of your life, you must practice and become masterful at making your preferences known to people as you engage in new friendships, work relationships and love interests.

Stop Looking For Approval

This third key point will give you permission internally to be yourself and let others know your preferences. Just remember that it is more important to be respected than liked. This does not make you a mean person. You can set your preferences with others in a way that is firm, yet tactful and polite.

Embrace Change

Change is good if it leads you toward healing and a better life. Change is often uncomfortable in the beginning. Ultimately, it must be accomplished to evolve. You can begin with small things you know need change and work up to larger issues. For instance, you may change your living environment at first. The simple task of cleaning out closets and selling or donating things you do not need is actually a holistic way to begin healing internally. You are cleaning, clearing and making way for something better. You are getting rid of things that no longer serve you. Doing this on a physical level often leads to accomplishing the same on a mental level as well.

Fear

Last, do not fear rejection from others because you have limits. Their attempt to reject you over such a thing is a form of manipulation. You do not need that kind of friend, boss or lover. Instead, you need to hold your course with this and eventually attract people and situations to you that match the level of self-worth you now display daily.

Journal or Writing Exercise:
When you are attracting people or situations you do not want, ask questions like:

- What am I feeling inside?
- What mood dominates me now?
- What can I do to set my preferences in this situation?
- What do I fear?
- How can I find balance?

By analyzing, you can begin finding solutions. Explore these questions any way that makes you feel comfortable. You can write and journal about your feelings and impressions. You can draw or a combination of the two. Just look deep as you can at all aspects and allow yourself to feel.

To summarize this chapter, when you work on setting and instituting preferences, you are building your inner power. This means you are entering a state where you do not sabotage yourself. By moving yourself forward, you are able to craft your life in a beautiful way that feeds your soul. Grow your inner power by continually looking within at the shadow side of yourself. After you have seen what needs to be remedied, take action to make sure it is followed through upon. As an abuse survivor who is going to fully bloom into your best self, you must be confident standing in your power — not allowing others to manipulate because you did not have clear preferences or boundaries.

All of this can seem like a very tall mountain to climb. Where do you begin? One step at a time. Soon, you look back and see the old you that was so fearful that you were allowing others to not only run your life, but ruin it too. With your preferences in place, there will be no question in the mind of others that you are a courageous person who feels a real sense of self worth. You are a person who will not be taken advantage of and this shows you really care about yourself which you so richly deserve.

12 – Reconnecting

As a child and teen, we cannot wait to grow another year older, celebrating not only our birthday, but inching forward toward being a grown up. Somehow in our child-like brains, we thought being on this grown up level would bring immense satisfaction we were missing out on. Once we became adults, we would not have to follow rules and have people tell us what to do, or so we thought. We would live each day however we wanted. We did not realize that once we could drive, we would also experience car repairs, high insurance bills and even being in vehicular accidents. We did not realize that we would have to follow rules to get money and listen to bosses we didn't like just to pay for the privilege of owning and driving a vehicle. We had no concept of what it would be like to sit with no electricity because we didn't pay the bill. Once adulthood was thrust upon us, some would find they needed to run back to the safety of parental figures for help.

Why were we in such a hurry? For some, it was the abusive conditions at home that made us want to flee. For others, it was the act of being able to say we were an adult. We were much too anxious to give up the good parts as well, to call ourselves that. As adults, if we decide to reconnect with those wonderful child like qualities we have buried inside, it is transforming to us on every level: mental, physical and spiritual.

Reconnecting with our child part, that free and true being who came into this world with nothing holding them back, is essential for inner fulfillment and lasting peace. It further propels us toward a purpose in life that gives our hearts and minds meaning. When we engage in activities some may see as only for children, at times we receive criticism. Ignore others who say these activities are wasteful or irrelevant. Often, these things are ways you are healing your inner child.

When I was in my early twenties, I began taking formal dance classes again in ballet and jazz. I went to class with a compelling need to do this for my body. After all, I had left my body and stayed in my mind way too long after my sexual abuse. I would leave the class in a hurry, feeling guilt for indulging in this once per week activity because it seemed trivial and close family members did see it that way. My finances were not so great and it was a monetary expense I did not need to take on. But, it brought me joy and reconnection with my physical body. At the time, I had not had therapy since right after the abuse. I did not know at the time that it also served to help heal my inner child and her needs.

Holistically, dancing grounds us and gives each of our muscles joy to move and stretch in ways we are not ordinarily moving. It pumps oxygen to our brains, allowing us to switch our focus on each body movement in a coordinated fashion that can be memorized or not. If you are in physical condition to move your body through sequenced or even free style dancing, I highly recommend this as a way to not only lighten your mood, but reconnect with your inner child-like nature.

Many survivors incorporate yoga as not only exercise, but a way of reconnecting with their self and higher God Source. Yoga can be hard on those who have allowed themselves to become stiff in the joints or have a weakened system in general. If you find yourself in that condition but still want to try yoga, consider finding an instructor or online video that caters to older adults practicing this art. This is often referred to as gentle yoga. This way, you can achieve the yoga benefits and work your body in a slower manner. In the United States, most YMCA's have a Silver Sneakers class for older adults for movements of this sort.

Another consideration is Tai Chi. This ancient moving art form assists you in achieving balance in your energetic field as you make your way through slow, but deliberate movements. It is easy to find video instruction on Tai Chi. Generally, you will be taken through a series of movements that serve to strengthen the entire energetic field and also assist you in feeling composed and at peace.

Qi Gong (pronounced chee gong) is another ancient body movement practice you may find very beneficial. Unlike tai chi, qi gong can be utilized to treat one area of the body you may be feeling stuck in or having trouble with. This practice can also be very beneficial for abuse survivors when used on any portion of the physical body, mind or spirit that needs assistance. It is a more focused type of Tai chi. Notice that both of these body movements contain the life force (Qi or chi). They are energy movements that help humans on every level, with qi gong focusing on specific areas.

Sitting or walking in nature instantly assists us in transforming our moods and dropping our minds into a more hypnagogic state. If you live near a park, forest, canyons, lakes, ocean or a botanical garden, love yourself by taking a short trip there often. Find a place where you feel safe. If you need company, bring along a friend. You may want to experiment with not speaking to each other while on your walk or journey into the beautiful area you have chosen. The more you keep your mind in a state to converse, the harder it will be to have what I like to term a walking meditation. And if you are unable to walk, sitting in your chosen area is just as beneficial. This is a quiet time when you soak in the smells, sights and sounds around you. Dogs can often be ideal companions for these nature visits.

When you have found some favorite nature spots to visit, think about bringing along a journal or sketchbook. You could also use the recording feature on your phone. Ideas will come to you at times. They are often important and can help speed your recovery toward your best life. Capture these ideas even if they seem impossible or silly at the time.

All of these ideas above move you toward reconnecting with your original essence — the real you that arrived on this planet on your birthday. This is the "you" that has so much potential, but was thwarted in its growth and development from those that sought to control it.

Inner Child

We are not repeating the past or moving backward when we work on healing our inner child. Instead, we are slipping back to make something right that was wronged in our past. By doing this, we actually propel ourselves forward in our healing journey. Even if your sexual abuse occurred as an adult, there are many walking around with a wounded inner child. Let's explore healing this precious being that is part of you.

Many of you were abused, exploited or hurt during this time of your life. Your focus will be to bring your inner child out of the shadows and help them feel loved and valued just for who they are.

When my first therapist wanted me to explore my inner child, I thought it was sort of silly. I really did not see any significance with it. So, just like journaling initially, this was another thing I resisted, making my recovery and healing longer than it needed to be. However, there are times when we are not ready for certain concepts. That is always acceptable. You must heal in your own way and time.

It has been said that, as children, our brains stay most of the time in a theta wave mode. Theta ranges from 3 to 8 Hz in measurement. This state resembles how one feels when having a deep daydream, meditating or the slow brain state we find ourselves in as we fall asleep or just as we awake. Theta wave state is very healing for the brain and therefore benefits the body as well. The theta state has also been described as experiencing things from within instead of being led by external stimuli. It is an ideal state for a type of learning that is more akin to gnosis. It can also be a very intuitive and receptive state.

I believe that children vacillate between theta and alpha most of the time. In the alpha state, we are more aware of our present surroundings and receptive to learning about what is right in front of us.

I bring up the brain wave states for two reasons. First, because children are primarily operating in these slower, deeper states, any trauma experienced during childhood can greatly affect them. The second reason I bring up brain states is that I want you to become more aware of yours. This will assist you in knowing how you are processing things at any given time.

Children can carry emotional wounds from all kinds of things, not just sexual abuse. Neglect, as well as verbal, physical and emotional abuse is damaging. Being abandoned by a parent or caregiver is significant. It all affects our inner child.

Part of our healing journey is to write a new story just for us. This helps us create our new life. However, many times we bump up against old things that seem to be preventing us from having that new life. Almost always … it has something to do with our inner child.

When we were children and found ourselves in our unique situation growing up, we had to learn how to survive and be part of the family group we were in. You could have had the most wonderful parents, but they berated you when you did certain things. You quickly learned that was not acceptable and if you wanted to be part of the family, you had to conduct yourself in a certain manner. That would be a mild thing for inner child wounding, but could be carried over into someone's adult life by having a lack of confidence or not accepted for your differences from others.

Some children learned to stay invisible. That meant not bothering their parents. Mom, dad (or both) were wrapped up in their own concerns and really not there for the kids. This made it hard for that child to speak up and ask for what they wanted. Feeling wanted was difficult. A child in this situation might even act out in some manner in order to gain attention. This also can carry over into our adult lives.

Children need to be valued for who they are, given the right kinds of attention and help with learning new things. When parents cannot or will not be there for them, they begin to feel like they do not count or matter. This can be played out in a number of ways as they grow up and it can continue into adulthood all the way to old age.

With only those few examples, you can get an idea of how we, as adults, can still be acting out our inner child's wounds on a consistent basis. It might mean we lack confidence, hold certain fears, do certain things for attention, or just walk around not feeling good enough.

When we do not feel loved or safe as children, this carries over into adulthood. Some children were not believed about abuse they endured or were too frightened to talk about it. This can set up a dynamic in our adult lives that keeps us from having our needs met --- as if we do not count. For children who were sex trafficked, their now adult counterpart can begin to think their only value as adults is to give others pleasure, seduction or money.

Many adults carry shame with them like an invisible cloak. Because, you see ... we carry that child with us all the time. And there is only one way to pacify it. It is for you to be the mother or father to it that it deserves. To be the parent it never had – the parent who can give the inner child what it needs to heal from its trauma and wounds. What happens if we do not heal our wounded inner child? Several things can happen.

Some people try to make the inner child feel better by overspending and buying lots of things. This sets up a vicious cycle with their budget and finances, often putting them into bankruptcy. Some people acquire other addictions to calm their inner child. This could be alcohol, drugs, food, sex or any activity they engage in too much to where they know it is out of balance and hurting, not helping them. Those items are really just the tip of the iceberg. Most of the time, we see it in failed relationships with the wrong kinds of people. Inner child issues can show up in the confidence and creativity in which we approach our life.

It is worth trying to help this wounded child inside of ourselves. I would love for you to consider engaging in this activity. Find a photo of yourself as a child – a small picture is ideal. Put it in a location where you will see it often such as taped to a mirror, held by a magnet on your refrigerator, taped to the side of your computer screen – somewhere you will see it frequently.

Each day, look at the photo and say with meaning: "I love you." As days go on, say new things to your inner child. Tell them how beautiful or handsome they are, how smart, funny or any other things that come to mind about this child. Become a champion for your inner child. Let it know that you, as the adult, will protect it and keep it safe. Let your inner child know you hold no judgments about it and that you think they are wonderful. Because, they are!

Work in your individual or group therapy with this concept of healing your inner child. Even if your sexual abuse did not occur until you reached adulthood, you still may have a wounded inner child that needs love, attention and the assurances of safety.

An idea shared by one therapist was to allow my inner child to write a letter to me about their feelings and life. This was very revealing and pretty emotional. I remember that I actually stayed home taking the day off work. I looked at old photos of my childhood and teen years. I read cards and letters from my family. After allowing my inner child to tell me how she had been feeling for years, I realized so much. Of course, there were obvious things I knew she would tell me. But, there were also some elements of her that I found surprising. Additionally, she was funny and endearing. She wanted to come out of hiding. She wanted to be loved just for who she was.

I suggest that you do this when you have alone time, of course. You may also do it within a therapy setting. Realize that you could become very emotional during this. Just like a child would write something, do not worry about spelling or sentence structure. Just let the inner child share their thoughts with you on how they are hurt or what they feel they are missing.

This process can be very healing because your inner child has truths it wants to reveal to you. It wants to step out of the shadows and be heard without judgment or any fear involved. With that in mind, you want to hold a special place for this child part of you that they can rest assured is safe. Allow this child to reveal feelings – perhaps even images. You may want to gaze at your photo while connecting with your inner child like this. Share this work with those you are in therapy with if you wish for clarification.

Persons who are still being abused, who are emotionally distressed, or have thoughts of harming someone or themselves should not engage in this without consulting a licensed professional in the field of psychology. The reason is that we have so much at the root of our child beginnings. For many, this brings up deep wounds that need attention immediately.

I also do not want to instill fear about it. I just want you to take stock of your current state before embarking on it alone. Use caution, however, when beginning to bring your inner child out of the shadows. Sometimes they are very hurt and angry. Working with your inner child is a very worthwhile endeavor and it can absolutely bring you considerable insights and speed your healing process.

Consider also – maybe a couple of times per month or once per week, doing something that is spontaneous, but safe, and perhaps childlike. Maybe there was a sport, activity or something you wanted to do as a child or teen that you were blocked from doing. Now, might be a good time to consider something like this for you and your inner child.

Perhaps you always wanted a certain item for your birthday that never came. You could gift it to yourself now. There is nothing wrong with that. Do something for your inner child in an area where they felt deprived of something.

You can make much progress when doing the inner child work and it might be something that is ongoing for you for awhile. If you cannot allow your inner child to speak by writing to you right now, at least just try posting a photo of yourself where you will see it often and remember to tell that child how much you love it.

Voice of The Inner Child

Children are often told to be silent about many things. From a young age, they are indoctrinated at school to be quiet. Any teacher knows that they cannot allow chaos to rule in their classroom. Yet, this silencing of children who have been sexually abused is rampant. In fact, young teen children and adults are also silenced in many ways. Often, we do not speak out because we are afraid of the reactions of others. Yet, it is so important to bloom that you give yourself a voice to do just that. By growing and being strong in knowing what you may come up against when you speak, you can overcome so many things. Knowledge is power to make changes.

One of the most harmful forms of abuse that survivors come up against is invalidation. This form of psychological abuse is so subtle. Often, we don't recognize we are enduring it. At times, we are perpetrating it upon ourselves because somewhere along the way in our life, we have been taught to do this. In fact, invalidation is pervasive in our world.

Invalidation occurs when people minimize, dismiss or reject the story or experiences of others. They discount their feelings, sometimes relating that they need to just toughen up. This is especially true with male survivors. Yet, there are many statements made to dismiss abuse that survivors have experienced.

Invalidation occurs when a victim comes forward and people do not believe them or want to minimize their experience. It probably took a ton of courage for that person to speak about their situation. If they are invalidated by others, it can make them wish they could crawl into a corner and hide. Invalidation is psychological abuse and mistreatment. At times, it can even make survivors doubt their own sanity.

From the beginning of my rescue, I was thrust into situations where it did not feel safe to talk about it. This was in the 1970's and I would hope that conditions are different now. Much of it could depend upon what part of the world we are speaking of. But, I was not just rescued from my perpetrators. I was arrested. The officer that booked me at the police station made a point of telling me I was a very bad little girl for the things I had participated in. As they transported me to a juvenile facility and put me in solitary confinement, no one explained anything. No one asked me anything. It felt like no one cared. I wanted to kill myself so much that night and for some nights thereafter.

Once my relatives drove out of state to pick me up at the juvenile facility, the car ride home was terribly quiet. No one talked. There was just silence. I suppose in my mind this made it unsafe to speak of what had happened to me. I am sure my family did not know what to say to me. I am also sure I was too ashamed to begin speaking of my experiences. So, the situation fit fine for all of us. Their silence sort of invalidated what happened and mine did as well. Everything around me, however, was feeling like I could not speak up for myself with anyone. I had been raped, trafficked, drugged and abused.

Fifteen years later, I took the initiative to begin therapy on my own. At around the age of thirty, I was invalidated by two people in my life for trying to get help. I was told untruths about therapy and how it did not help. My sociopath boyfriend said it was just a money making endeavor and self-indulgence. A relative said I was just drudging up old stuff and needed to forget about it and go on with my life. Did they know I was feeling suicidal at times? Here is the secret about both of these individuals. Therapy taught me how much I needed to stay away from them. Their personalities were toxic and harmful. Perhaps at a certain level, they knew that could be a result. My advancement in therapy or with self help would reveal who they really were and give me the confidence to break free from them.

I forged ahead with therapy plus working on my own with every self-help book I could read that interested me. I listened to guided meditations and motivational material from some of the giants in the industry. My sociopath boyfriend told me those endeavors were nonsense as well. I finally realized one evening after breaking my ankle in two spots ice skating with him that the relationship had to end forever. As he drove my car to the hospital (since my right ankle was no longer working) he repeatedly berated me for crying in pain. He said I probably just sprained my ankle and was nothing more than a big baby. He invalidated my experience. There I was with broken bones – one completely shattered – and he was not going to accept this as the reality I was experiencing. He did not want to deal with my inconvenient pain.

As survivors, our experiences and stories are often inconvenient for others. They don't know what to do or how to respond to tales of abuse. Instead, they would rather sweep it under the rug.

Sometimes, we will find people – perhaps many of them that invalidate our experience. This can happen in all kinds of ways. As we try to speak up and out about what happened to us at any age in our lives, they either do not believe it at all or they want to minimize its effect upon us. When this happens, it can leave us doubting ourselves. Without knowing it, these people are participating in this form of emotional abuse that psychologists have clearly recognized as psychological invalidation.

When others invalidate our experience, they are doing it for several reasons. Let's look at those so that we will not feel confused about the experience we are having or had in the past.

Most of those around us do not mean to do this, but some do. There are mean spirited people and you need to just steer clear of them. I see many of them on the Internet. It's easy for them to hide behind their electronic walls and project nasty bitterness to others. While I do not know what lies at the root of their negativity and cruel words, I suspect someone hurt them and they are dealing with it in this manner. Perhaps they feel if they lash out at others first, they will escape hurt.

Most people that invalidate our experience in one way or another are not cruel or mean. They could be in shock, denial and just don't want to believe things like this happen or at least not this close to them. This can make them want to reject the information entirely. There are many reasons for this. First, if the abuse occurred within a family, they might feel they suddenly are in a position of having to pick sides. I believe this is why we often hear of mothers not wanting to validate what their children are telling them about abuse they are enduring from a relative in the family. That relative could be a father, step-father, live in boyfriend, uncle, or even a sibling. Thrust into a position of having to believe this could be going on is going to rock everyone's world. Lines must be drawn and authorities brought in. Everything in life will change. It is easier to just remain in denial about this. And this is very tragic for the child involved. Not only do they not receive validation and a type of rescue that is needed, they are forced to continue living a lie. In most cases, the abuse continues. This can truly cause a mental split for them because the person who was supposed to love and defend them the most in this world, their mother, is denying their experience. Sadly, there are cases where the mother herself is the abuser.

Another way we see invalidation happen is through minimizing. By trying to make you think that it was not that bad, so far in the past, you should be over it now, and other such ideas. This type of invalidation clearly does not allow you, as someone who endured abuse, to have feelings that need to be expressed and healed.

And then there is the silent treatment where people pretend you did not reveal your closely guarded secrets to them, even though you did. This can be quite devastating. They may give you the silent treatment or just walk away and leave you. When a young person experiences this, it leaves them feeling helpless. When an older person has this happen, it can make them feel guilty for sharing. All of a sudden, they feel as if they crossed a line with someone who does not want to know about their real life and experience. Instead, they want to keep everything on the surface and not go into those deeper waters. This is tragic because it is these experiences that can create very unique bonds between you and others who are willing to listen in a non-judgmental way and also acknowledge your story.

Thankfully, in many places in the world, you are able to seek out vocal expression of your pain or experience through individual and group therapy. That is a safe place where you should not encounter invalidation.

Ironically, one of the worst perpetrators of invalidation can be you. I spent many years doing this – saying to myself that I just needed to forget and move on and never allowing myself to feel what I needed to in order to heal. As survivors, we must always know in our heart that our feelings matter. In fact, we should be checking in with ourselves often about how we are feeling. When we have tools in place that help us in coping, this really advances our ability to forge ahead in life and heal.

Invalidation is one of our largest fears because almost all of us have already experienced its damaging effects. Psychological invalidation sets up patterns in our subconscious where we can begin to put our feelings and needs aside as if they don't matter as much as the needs of others.

When you look at your life right now, are there areas where you invalidate yourself? Are there things you need to do for you that are not getting done because you have relegated them as not that important? This is part of patterns we slip into when we have experienced more than our fair share of psychological invalidation.

And if you are currently seeking help, therapy or validation in any form and people are engaging in this with you, I urge you to break away from them or make a big stand. This is like someone trying to ignore that you have a broken leg. Are you going to go along with them that your leg is not broken? Of course not, because the pain is too great. Yet when it comes to our psychological pain, the items that cannot be seen, it is easy for others to invalidate our experience. We must stand up and not allow this – one way or another. Those who want to manipulate you to cover for their own bad behavior tell their victims they are crazy, too sensitive, or worse … lying.

If our abuse happened prior to adulthood, this often silences our inner child. All abusers of children use invalidation to manipulate. This can be parental figures that are verbally or physically abusive. It does not have to involve sexual abuse. Once the abuser engages in psychological invalidation with the child, they have added this type of emotional abuse to their list of wrong deeds.

When we look at psychological invalidation, most of us have been experiencing this since childhood in one form or another. It is up to us to give a voice to our inner child. We can do this through many mediums – speaking, journaling, writing, singing, art and music. Your inner child needs to be heard. Only you can be the champion for this child. And when they speak, do not silence him or her with invalidation. Whatever your inner child feels is valid. Their perception of events is valid. It needs to be heard.

Invalidation is what has made you feel briefly at times that the thoughts you hold about your memories are not real. This is the way invalidation works like a virus eating away at us inside.

What can be done? First, recognize when this is going on with others. That is the most important step – knowledge. Also, acknowledge when it is going on with you. How are you invalidating your own feelings, physical, educational, financial or emotional needs? Once you start seeing these patterns, a light is shown on this dark shadowy essence that you could not identify before.

The next thing you can do is acquire developed responses when anyone attempts to invalidate you. Here are some ideas and they all begin with the word "I" and involve you stating how you feel. Just remember that. For instance,

"I do not feel believed."

"I feel judged."

"I feel as if your silence is because you do not want to know my situation."

You could even say, "I feel as if I am being invalidated."

Try not to blame them directly as this tends to close down the conversation. With some personality types, it will send them on the attack. Many of you will just want to shut down and not deal with the invalidation. Some of you will want to confront people doing this in an accusatory or aggressive manner. Both of these methods are lower on the list of fruitful ways to handle it. But, at least it is being handled.

The Wounded Inner Child

Would you hand car keys to a child? In my book, *Dreaming Synchronicity*, I have a short interlude where I tell of a dream I had while writing the book. The memoir was going to reveal many of my secrets including those of my sexual abuse. The dream, in many ways, encapsulated many of my fears. Dreams give us glimpses into ourselves by showing us things that are symbolic or archetypical. Significant personal growth can be gained by analyzing the dreams we remember.

In the dream, there was a young girl I was trying to appease. I recognized her (after the dream) as representing my inner child. She had been following me around during the busy dream I was having. In fact, she almost felt attached to me. Feeling that her presence was hindering me, I placed her in a vehicle with two other young girls to watch a children's movie so that I could focus on my tasks without her distraction. Of course, in order to do this, I had to leave the keys in the car so that the movie could play in the vehicle off the car's battery. She started the car and began backing it up. I stopped her and then fixed the vehicle so the movie would play without the keys present. In other words, I stopped her from taking control of the vehicle because she is not experienced as a driver or old enough to drive. Now, what this represents is many things.

My inner child is acting out and trying to take control in situations that are too adult for her. She was also tugging on my apron strings (so to speak) constantly following me. She wanted to be heard and her story told.

My intervention in keeping her from controlling the vehicle was to keep her and the other girls from harm. You can read much into this as I see myself as one who wants to help and protect children. Yet, I have learned over time that our inner child possesses a key that we, as the adult, may have overlooked. The inner child can be thought of as the new young human we came into this world as. The young soul who experienced certain conditioning and happenings that later colored and affected their grown up adult counterpart.

One of the reasons that we explore the inner child and healing that portion of us is so that we can bring out our true inner self – the self that would have been whole. Due to our upbringing and things that happened to us during childhood, it still affects us as adults.

An inner child or what you may have experienced during childhood will impact you in your adult life, especially if you endured trauma. A child that has been traumatized by neglect or abuse of any kind carries wounds that need to be healed. We have the power to do this for ourselves

When people hear the term wounded child, they imagine an adult who has gone to the edge with violence, crimes against others, etc. And, this is something that can and does happen with many who carry this unhealed wounded child. Yet, the wounded child also appears in much more subtle ways that affect a person's life.

Sometimes I see the wounded child that we may have within ourselves as a quiet little mouse that is continuing to have babies and multiply. We don't even know it is in our house. When our adult life is not shining the way we want it to, in ways it could be, we often need to look at this inner child. If everything you are trying to do to improve your life through your vocation, career, education, physical health, appearance or relationships is not working or too challenging, look to the past with the inner child.

By looking back to the patterns of childhood you can see what is holding you back. Patterns developed at a young age can be invisible to you like the mouse. Yet, they grow and multiply. Over time, you can become very dissatisfied or confused with your life because you do not know how to correct it.

Worse, we can see that over generations, adults who never effectively deal with their own childhood wounds often repeat these cycles of abuse, fear, violence, neglect, poverty and addictions. At the very least, they often repeat and teach beliefs to their children that are not really grounded in truth, but in a system of ideas they adopted from their own upbringing.

Some of the things we see ourselves doing can be things like bottling up our emotions because when we were children it was not safe to express how we felt, whether it was sadness, grief, anger, jealousy or any other feeling that a parental figure did not want to deal with.

Some of us find it hard to speak our truth and give a voice to ourselves because as a child, we were silenced in one way or another. Therefore, we find it hard in adult life to speak up and state our preferences or confront those who do us wrong or do not respect our boundaries.

Many adults fail to establish boundaries with others because somewhere in childhood they received the message that their needs do not matter as compared to the needs of others around them. In their adult life, they now have a difficult time setting up their own preferences and rules of engagement with others because they fear being rejected, criticized or abandoned if they do.

It is not uncommon for feelings of anger, bitterness or anxiety to be a symptom of needing to heal the inner child. It can also show up as a lack of confidence or low self-worth. We may have fears of being abandoned, alone or trusting people in general. Many abuse survivors suffer bouts of feeling safe at different times and places. We are unknowingly repeating patterns that are held within from childhood or adolescence.

Does our inner child hold a key to unlock many of the repetitive patterns we see in our adult life that are not working well for us? And if this inner child does have the key, how can we as adults, get them to turn it over to us so that we can unlock the door and experience our world with more confidence and positive experiences?

First, we need to befriend this child or adolescent and become familiar with it once more. We must almost begin a new relationship with this part us that has hidden itself in the shadows of our psyches.

How can we cultivate a rich and rewarding experience for the child inside us? What do we need to think about or do differently in order to achieve that? Let's begin with what all children want to experience so that we can know where we need to make adjustments.

All children want to feel loved and appreciated just for their pure existence. And, they should be. They want to be praised and encouraged. Children crave attention and want to be verbally rewarded. They want to be told, I love you. They want to be told how good and smart they are.

When they make a mistake, they do not need to be shamed, discounted or made to feel stupid. They are children. They are learning and if we are good teachers, we would never do that. Instead, we would show them another way to achieve their objective. We would let them know it is okay to make mistakes and that is a natural part of life and learning. If we are not making some mistakes, we are not reaching and trying to do something different.

Children want to know we are there for them – that we will protect them from harm and take care of their human needs such as food, shelter, education, etc. Children can carry emotional wounds from all kinds of thing. Neglect, as well as verbal, physical and emotional abuse is damaging. Being abandoned by a parent or caregiver is significant. It all affects our inner child.

When we do not feel loved or safe as children, this carries over into adulthood. Some children were not believed about abuse they endured or were too frightened to talk about it. This can set up a dynamic in our adult lives that keeps us from having our needs met — as if we do not count. We carry that child with us all the time. And there is only one way to pacify it. It is for you to be the mother or father it deserves. To be the parent it never had – the parent who can give the inner child what it needs to heal from its trauma and wounds.

Here is the thing: you need to identify how the beautiful child or adolescent in you is hurting. You need to know how this hurt can be healed. This is so individualized that I strongly urge you to explore this with a trained counselor or psychological professional. Having this other trained person there to bounce things back to you that perhaps you cannot see will help you immensely. Plus, they can provide many tools that will speed your wounded child recovery.

As you begin to explore methods and tools for helping your wounded inner child, if any of these exercises are too emotionally painful for you, please come back to them at another time when you feel stronger. Perhaps when you are further along on this healing journey, you can attempt again. As stated earlier, much of exploring the wounded child is best done with psychological support help from trained professionals. Many of you have endured horrific abuse during your child or teen years. These emotions and feelings that arise from the dark can often put you in a position where you need a trained person there to help you through. If you feel like you can do one or more of these exercises on your own, by all means go ahead and give it a go.

My first method for discovering what key the inner child holds for us to open the door and know what is going on inside is fairly simple. Take a piece of paper or journal and contemplate this:

Write about your placement in the family of origin you grew up in and how it made you feel. I don't want to lead you too much through this because I want your thoughts and feelings to be your own. However, an example could be that you grew up as a middle child. You may have felt like you had to compete for attention from the first child or the baby of the family below you. Or, you could be the first child and have always felt like you had to be responsible for everyone else.

I was a first child born to a young teen mother. I have considered it my duty to make others feel good my entire life. I see how this happened from childhood. At times, I had to comfort or help her and I did that, because I was a sensitive, empathetic child. I soothed her if she had a fight with my father and I stood beside her as tears streamed down her face and wiped them away. In many ways, I learned mothering from a young age and I have spent considerable time struggling with codependency issues because of it.

Conversely, my father wanted me to learn things and be smart. Being pretty was nice but it was very important to be intelligent. It was also very important that I was a free thinker. These were positive things for the most part. The most negative thing my father taught me was to ignore my feelings. This is because he ignored his. But, I couldn't. I was such a feeling, empathic child that it was difficult at that young age. As I accumulated traumas going forward, I did begin to stuff those feelings deep inside of all that had transpired. But, that is another long story. My point is that some of the simple ways we grew up within our family of origin can be affecting us long into adulthood in the ways we act and respond to others around us, including ourselves. It can even show in the way we carry ourselves – something that other people observe about us.

This exercise will begin to show you how your inner child may respond to life and how that part of you feels their placement in life is affected. If other thoughts arise from your inner child and their feelings at this time, go ahead and journal those as well. You can take this exercise as far as you feel comfortable. The point of it, of course, is to uncover the hidden ideas and beliefs you accumulated from your upbringing and experiences. How have they affected you? Does it color the way you see your life? Does it affect the way you are treated by others?

Exercise number two is going to shock you when you do it. You are going to really begin to hear who is controlling you. For this, you will need a notebook. It can be small enough to fit in your purse or pocket. That is probably best because you will carry it with you for awhile. You could also use a small voice recorder or the app on your phone to record. Here is what to do:

Each time you have a voice in your head that tells you that you are not capable, cannot do something, not good enough or any other combination of these types of thoughts, I want you to record it or write it down. Do this for three days and be diligent as you can about it. You are going to be amazed (as I was) how many times you knock yourself down. It does not matter how long you have been practicing positive thoughts or have been on a personal growth or healing journey – you still have these thoughts and you will be surprised at their frequency.

Don't try to keep track of these negative things going on in your head instead of writing them down. This is not a memory exercise. This is a technique for you to uncover and see patterns. Once you see these underlying patterns that are unknowingly affecting your life, you can correct them.

Knowing who we are is critical. We discover that by doing the work of healing the inner child. Many of us do not take proud ownership of talents and skills we have. Instead, we always feel it is not good enough. This is a parental voice speaking inside that told us we need to try more, do better, cannot possibly accomplish this or that. Come to know and love your gifts. Cultivate them more. When you do, you can be more comfortable in your skin.

Last, but not least, continue talking to the photo of yourself as a child or teen each day. That image of yourself should be placed somewhere you will see it often. Tell that child how you know it has hurt and you are listening to it now. Tell that child you love it and how happy you are that it is making itself known to you.

The Magical Child

Healing your inner child can assist you in uncovering the magic elixir that exists in each of us at the beginning of life.

In our world, there is always uncertainty. This can be such a damper on your spirit. It can hold you back from accomplishing in life. And, it is this uncertainty, along with the negative words projected by others, that really keeps us from being our best selves. Another item that can keep us from feeling the same type of lively excitement a child does is a mundane existence. We need to sometimes vary the things we routinely do to make things a little more spontaneous.

The other day, I was working on a deadline with another person, assisting them in research for their project. I finally realized after a couple of hours that I really needed to break away and do something totally creative and more right brain in nature – an activity where I did not have to think so much. It made all the difference to do this. Once I gave my brain that needed break, I was able to go back and approach the project in a robust manner that saw it to completion. In fact, I have already scheduled three weeks off from writing and book production once this book is complete and published. During that time, I will be working on actively marketing this work. However, I plan to spend a portion of my free time creating other things in my craft room — a place I have not visited for months. I am sure there will be more than a few cobwebs to clear before I begin and always I seem to need to reorganize things before I begin working on a project.

If I am lucky, perhaps I will go away for a few days with my husband to have some solace and alone time for us. This me time is critical to refilling my creative well. I realize that not everyone has the luxury of doing this. Believe me, neither did I for years. Yet, somehow I managed to play at something as a hobby or activity that brought me great satisfaction even if it was only for a short time.

As children, we gravitated toward playing with things that gave us the most satisfaction in the moment – whatever was available. A child can find the oddest things to have fun with. They will create things with dirt or cardboard boxes. Store bought toys lie in wait while they turn the most common things into creations of their imagination. Their imagination is active and they are able to work magic by turning their current existence into something else entirely just with the power of their minds. But they also have another superpower. Once they are preoccupied and engaged, children are doing this (especially young ones) without concern about how the play will end or what their art project will turn into. They are delighted in the process, very much in the moment and focused on inner satisfaction and joy from the creative play.

This is the magical aspect of being a child. And, it is this child we need to love and cultivate in order to soften the hard edges we have accumulated during our time "growing up". The sole benefit we have in nurturing, reconnecting with and hearing our inner child – especially the one who is wounded, is that we can finally break free and live a fuller life. We begin to find our purpose.

I remember when I was in the world of business that when my family took a vacation, I was really struggling the first two to three days of the holiday to relax and just be in that moment. Instead I was worried about what was going on with my business. I remember one beach vacation where I actually brought along a fax machine … just in case I had contracts I needed to sign. I realized this about myself and my husband was carrying his business mind on the trip with him also. We just could not seem to relax the first few days, despite the fact that we were both very excited to be on vacation and in the location we chose. This inability to leave the concerns of adulthood behind meant we were taking life much too serious. We were not making room for play. Before we left home, we had imagined ourselves having fun and doing various things that were more childlike. Thankfully, we would eventually relax and be in total vacation mode.

I know many people like this. We do this out of habit. It can also be a fear or a sense that this is where our ego or personality exists – in this adult world of worries. In our minds, we are this adult person who must be available to take care of important grown up things. How can we suddenly transform into a person who frolics around on the beach. But, that's who we need to be. That is a part of reconnecting with our inner child.

Here is another thing to consider. During the time we are wrapped up in our business career minds or adult modes, we can easily be fooled into thinking that is who we really are. The real truth is that as you connect with your inner child, you discover the real you – the human that you came into this planet as. By uncovering the aspects of your pure original self, you fall in love more with yourself. You are appreciating you for who you truly are instead of the titles or occupation you hold in life. You are not born a mother or father. You are not born a nurse, carpenter, assembly line worker, artist, or CEO. These are just things you might do for awhile, things you might be for a time period or might adopt. Or even in the case of parenthood, have happen to you.

You also were not born a victim. You were not born that. Even if you were victimized as an infant or toddler, you were not born that way. That is not the true you ... anymore than you were born with a suit and tie on and going into the office each day. You were born as an individual who had certain traits and talents inherent in you. This is true just as much as you were born with brown, green, blue or hazel eyes. You are not what you think you are much of the time. The real you is the one with all the potential that came into this world. Reconnecting with your inner child and healing their wounds will help you find that.

On a deep level, whatever we achieve or become in life are just trappings. They are wonderful and we should celebrate them, but what we believe we have become may not be the real person -- the real person we need to love inside at a very core level. As you heal and recover your inner child by doing the work, you understand yourself more and you know what you like and what works for you. As you know this, you set preferences (boundaries) for that child to say, "No, I'm sorry this relationship is not going to work." "No, this job is not going to work for me." You come out of victimhood by reconnecting and healing that inner child. As you do this, you gain confidence. You feel in your life that what you are doing is boosting the real you – revealing what you came here for. You begin to find your true purpose and follow it.

You also learn not to judge yourself so harshly because to do so would be critical of your inner child that lives within you. And you stay away from situations that you know may not be good for you – anything that may be considered toxic for sure. You avoid that to protect your inner child. All of this makes you feel more in control of yourself and your life, yet with a spontaneity and creativity that was not emerging before. It's like stepping into a new dimension that is more meaningful, deep, rich and beautiful. You set your life goals with excitement and purpose, but you don't feel like a failure if there are some you do not reach. You just readjust. You reexamine your goals and whether it is even still something you want to do or achieve. As you start living from this new frame of mind and the framework you are building as a foundation for yourself, things begin to come together and it makes life more fun and meaningful. We can all rediscover this child within us. By reconnecting with it and giving it the love and admiration it so deserves, we will live a more healed and magical life.

It is very important for you to stop feeling tainted or ruined in some way. Begin stating to yourself that you are perfectly imperfect and believe it. Say it with meaning in your mind and out loud. You are a piece of the creation that is learning and evolving. You are beautiful!

Imagine you work in a facility that produces paper. Your job is to take the raw materials and form specialized paper. Let's say you make watercolor paper. You have just created five new sheets of the specialty paper and you lay them aside. One is swept up by a sudden gust of wind and falls to the floor. In the meantime, another worker steps on that piece of paper without even knowing it and leaves a dark shoe print. You pick the piece of watercolor paper up and say, "Oh, too bad, this now goes to the reject pile."

As you put it in the reject pile, you realize that now you have accidently torn it on one corner. Now, it is further damaged. As it makes its way to the next stop in the factory, accountability must be made by another worker of why it ended up there. Someone writes on it "ruined not good for commercial sale". Think about this. That piece of paper began as perfect as the other four. It was created and existed with potential. Now, someone has stepped on it, someone has torn it and it has been judged to be not good enough for commercial sale and written on. All negative things – perhaps even traumatic events for the piece of paper. Pretend the paper has thoughts and feelings. What does it think of itself as it sits in the reject pile?

Yet, there is a person that loves to collect the paper that is not going to be sold. They want the paper that is considered imperfect. Being an artist and not having a lot of funds, this free paper comes in handy for them. They take the paper with the writing, shoe print and ripped corner and cut off the torn section, reducing the paper to the measurement they need for the piece they will create with it. They apply gesso to the shoe print and the writing and now have a blank canvas with which to create. Last, they begin their painting – something pleasing and wonderful for the senses. They create something that has meaning to them and to the person who will eventually purchase it and want to have it as their own. You see from this that they did not let the opinions of others determine the piece of paper was no longer any good. Instead, they saw the potential of it, made some modifications, and it turned out unique and beautiful.

What we know is that the wounded inner child benefits greatly from healing at some point. Otherwise, it becomes wrapped and integrated into the wholeness of what you are projecting out into the world. It affects how you are operating, showing what your core feelings are inside. That is because all of those things are there at a base level inside the brain. You have to realize this is all just stuff the piece of paper has experienced and endured. This is the writing, the tears and the footprints the paper has gone through. The piece of paper was created perfect originally. Along the way, things happened. But it does not mean that the piece of paper is worth less than the other paper it was created along side. What it means is that the paper is different and it can be celebrated for its differences. It can be enhanced in a way that its uniqueness shines something else to others. Remember that you are the artist of your own paper.

As survivors, it can be difficult to cultivate the magical child that already exists within us at first. This child has been thwarted – tapped down just like the lotus buried in the mud. All of the mental and emotional clearing spoke of heretofore in this writing leads you to the key that unlocks this. The actual work must be done and it is painful at times. Emotional clearing exercises and holistic helpers you choose can help your healing come about in a swifter manner.

Once you have cleared enough inner and outer debris by loving and taking care of your inner child, you must rediscover and ignite your inner fire. This will cause you to be more passionate about many aspects of your life. Children have exuberance and experience elation in the smallest things. Is it too late to rekindle that? There is laughter contained within passion.

Be confident and treat yourself well. Children are confident until it is undermined by others. Don't be one of the "others" to yourself. It is time to congratulate that child within you. Look at what they have come through. Notice how incredible they are. You are a work of art in motion.

Be inspired - find things that make you sing inside. When you were a child, just swinging on a swing set could make you relax and smile. There are so many things that make us feel better. Often, we refuse to do them and make the excuse of not having enough time or just don't feel like it. Hey, I understand. I do it too. Yet I always find that if I push through and make myself engage, I have a great time and gain much inspiration from it. Visit that museum to peruse the art work. Go to an amusement park or a movie. Walk in the rain and purposely take note of every small sound or thing you see visually. Childlike inspiration can be found alone, with someone else or in a group.

We lose a good portion of our childlike magic due to the programming we receive growing up. Our parents repeat the words and actions taught to them by their parents, most of it is unconscious. It does not stop with our parents. There are many sources of programming that tell us what we can or cannot do or be. Most of us grew up with television. There is a reason they call it television programming. That is what it is. From the shows we watch that tell us how to be a family unit to the news that regurgitates mostly the negative, we were and are still being programmed. Commercials told us constant messages: you can never be perfect enough, strong enough, clean enough, rich enough, beautiful enough. You are not enough. I hardly know anyone who does not have bouts of feeling like they may not be enough. Guess what? I am enough and so are you!

As we look through the lens of childhood, specifically of the inner magical child, we can see how life can take on a completely new direction and meaning. By spending time healing your inner child or adolescent – becoming their champion and best parent they could hope for in the world, you will unlock the door to integrating a magical child within yourself that keeps you vibrant, feeling young and whole for years to come. That is priceless to gift yourself and own.

Notes To Self

13 – Trust

When a caterpillar is encased within its cocoon, it has entered a dark introspective time in its life cycle. As humans, we also experience these dark times in our lives. They are always transformative on some level. The caterpillar trusts that it will survive, change and eventually be free and fly … something it could not do before. For us, we often are filled with tremendous self doubt when traveling through the more shadowing sides of our existence. Will we ever find what we are looking for in life? Will we be loved and able to fully love and trust another? Will we metaphorically be able to fly?

Trust is the bridge from dark times to lighter happier times. It contains the element of faith. It is common to find trust lacking within ourselves after experiencing trauma and betrayal at the hands of others. When this has occurred, especially surrounding sexual abuse, we unconsciously construct a grid around us to try and avoid anything like that from happening again. Often, we suspect others just because we lack trust. It could be they are a trustworthy human and we are misinterpreting things.

I know this about myself as one who endured that trauma. Decades later, I still catch myself sometimes in judging mode - trying to determine the true intentions of someone I know or have just met. Easy trust is elusive for me to place in others. I have found the strongest way I can relate happily in my world is to actively work on trusting myself.

Trust can become an unseen force when combined with personal faith and intention. Having a strong connection and belief in God Source has helped me tremendously as well. I am not going to lie to you. You are not simply going to read this chapter and all of a sudden have more trust of people, especially strangers. However, if you adopt the exercises I have built inside this writing and work at them through affirmations, notes to yourself, pop-ups on your computer screen, etc., you will find the steel grid around you begins to soften and become more pliable. It already has holes in it where others can see you and you can see them, but there has been a barrier there nonetheless that says, "Stop, I don't know if I can trust you."

What if you adopted a different idea about trust? Explore these concepts:

You trust that the sun will shine each morning, even if it is obscured by cloud cover. You know each day brings the sun. Likewise, you know that nightfall will happen. You trust that this will occur no matter what. Even if you live in the North Pole region, you are confident that long days with all sun and long nights with all darkness will end. The sun will shine again!

What other things could you feel this confident about? Look at this list and choose one or more to actively work on this month. Ideally, choose two — one that feels easy for you to trust and one that feels more difficult but that you would like to master.

I trust that my intuition is always available to me and I listen to its messages

I trust that all of my physical needs will be met

I trust that I can travel without accident or incident

I trust that even when things look or feel dark, there is light present and it will come to me

I trust that I will know which humans I can rely on and those I cannot because I have discernment

I trust that when I give of myself and my resources that I will always get back more than I gave

I trust my body to give me clues about what it needs to be in optimal state

I trust my mind to process, sort and give me information I need when I need it

I trust that as I work on myself and improve within, I find more joy and contentment

I trust that I set clear boundaries for those around me so that trust is not a big issue between us.

Road Blocks

There are so many reasons a sexual abuse survivor can experience trust issues. Many times you will run up against feelings that are difficult to sort out. In the beginning, it can be a challenge to discern whether you are experiencing paranoia or a true inner warning about some person or situation. It is important to realize that this happens with all people who have been betrayed by any form of abuse. That means it affects millions of people. Even if your abuser(s) were not in your own family, you may still experience trust issues with some of them. There are times when parents and/or siblings have let you down. Perhaps they revealed a confidence you wanted kept secret.

It is helpful to examine trust issues from the past. What was our part in these trust issues? We need to look at the "why". Why do we keep attracting people or situations which prove we cannot trust others? Perhaps the answer to this is very simple - we attract what we focus on the most. Feelings are what drive this train — not just thoughts. Therefore, if I am consciously or unconsciously walking around feeling as if all love relationships never work out — someone always cheats on the other, this is probably what I will experience because it is now a core belief. If I adopted an attitude that I am not good enough due to repeated abuse and that idea is sunk into my subconscious, I will certainly attract people who show me that is the case. We repeat what we do not repair. Depending upon the level of abuse you endured, this can take considerable time to work through.

Please do not misunderstand me. Anyone who breaks your trust is in the wrong and not off the hook. You are not to blame for their actions. The thing to look at here is how it can be prevented in the future. By asking yourself deep questions such as:

What is the primary mood or appearance I project to others? Is it one of being too nice? If so, realize that can allow many to feel they can walk all over you. Is it one of being too closed off? That can prevent you from experiencing meaningful exchanges and relationships with others. Do I trust people too easily without getting to know them for awhile? Examine this as you go about your daily life. Look at your part in the situation.

Without properly set boundaries and stating our preferences to others, we will always suffer from trust issues. Our inner child is begging us to be the adult who is not afraid to speak up and tell our truth, show what we will allow and what we will not.

Holistic Helpers

Rose quartz may be something you want to add either in a pendant worn or beside your bed as you sleep. This pink crystal helps to calm and balance the emotions and can even dissolve anger. Rose quartz is primarily linked with the fourth heart chakra. If you meditate with this gem on a regular basis, it can assist you in building inner trust. Combine it with labradorite or lapis lazuli to increase your intuition and discernment.

Love Relationships

Trust plays an integral part in all relationships. Finding enough trust to love someone in an intimate way is entirely possible after abuse. What are the main things you need to do in order to have a beautiful relationship?

1. Get to know the other person very well before having sex together. Sexual abuse survivors can often feel that sex is expected and rather soon after meeting someone. To some survivors, it is almost like shaking hands. Sex is one way some survivors feel validated about their very existence. The fact that another person desires you sexually can somehow be misconstrued to believe they actually care about you as a potential permanent partner. Perhaps this is true in rare situations. Most of the time, it is not. Sadly, the survivor can end up feeling hurt, abandoned, used and discarded.

When you are not meeting people for dating is a great time to set your preferences. How long is reasonable to get to know someone and what steps will you take to do that? Once you have laid ground rules, stick by them. Fantastic sex that is deeper and more meaningful easily happens when you develop a friendship first and allow things to evolve slowly.

2. Be friends first! This ties in with the getting to know each other. If you cannot have a very good friendship with this person, a long term relationship will not work. Review the chapter on Preferences to know what are normal requirements for friends and lovers.

3. Feel comfortable enough with this person that you can talk with them about any sexual concerns you have. Due to your abuse, certain things may turn you off or excite you. By developing this long term friendship, you will feel much freer to let your partner know why you may have some preferences in the bedroom.

4. Make any and all preferences known! Yes, you need to really make sure that you are not changing who you are to be who you think the other person needs. Have requirements and preferences. This is the highest form of loving you!

5. Make sure your preferences are respected and you respect theirs as well. When this does not happen, immediately talk and correct it.

6. Early in the getting to know them phase, analyze your attraction to this individual. Is there anything about the way they look or act that line up with a previous abuser? Review chapter 10.

7. Do not overindulge or perhaps indulge at all in alcohol or drugs that lower your barrier to keep things where they need to be during the getting to know each other phase. You know your body and limits.

As you read all of these strong suggestions above, you may think it takes all the fun out of things and contains no romance. I assure you romance, spontaneity and attraction can be achieved while you are dating and getting to know this individual. Your relationship will be built on a firmer foundation for long lasting success in all areas such as communication, loyalty and eventual sex with each other.

Last, if you find during the time you are getting to know this other person that they are not quite what you thought they were, you did the right thing by slowing it all down and not having sex. You will thank yourself and this is another way you have been a champion for your feelings and well being. It is a true sign of growth, healing and loving yourself enough not to give in to your first instincts. It shows true discipline.

Some sexual abuse survivors have endured situations that affected them so greatly they are traumatized by having sex later — even though it is something they are choosing with their own free will. This can occur in a number of ways including flashbacks, physical pain, emotional reactions and feelings of disgust. When this occurs, it compounds the need for a really good relationship based upon being true friends. When your partner is empathetic to your past and willing to work through this with you, great healing can happen. Spend time determining what makes you feel safer and grounded so that you can enjoy sexual relations together. Work on creating an understanding between the two of you on what items may trigger you.

Holistic helpers for feeling insecure sexually include flower essences of banana, iris and watermelon. Each of these essences assists to help dissolve barriers to connecting with your partner.

Notes To Self

PART II – Transforming With Nature

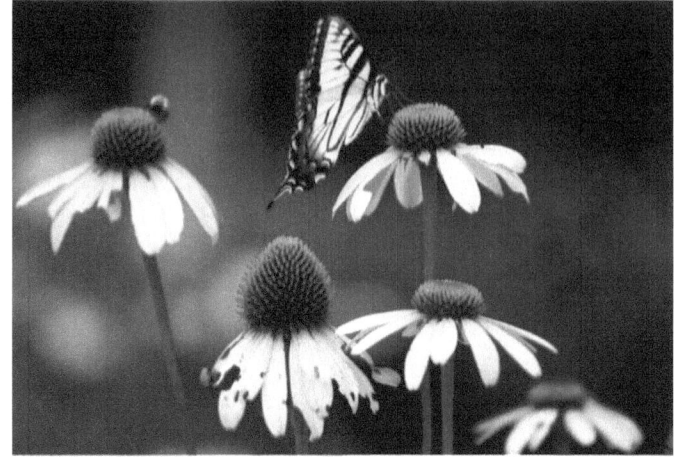

14 – Energy

Whether you personally know or believe it, everything is made of energy. Our physics now proves this hypothesis is true. While impossible to see with the human eye, something that seems very solid and stationary such as a rock or chair are made of tiny subatomic particles vibrating at a very fast rate. While we are all made up of these incredibly tiny energy particles, when you put certain people together, their energies can clash at times. We each carry our own energy signature, just as the plants, minerals and animals do. When it comes to flower essences, essential oils and herbs, each plant or flower carries its own individual essence or energy signature. Through trial and error, our use of these substances has evolved quite a bit. Some information has been received telepathically and passed on to others.

Over time, practitioners have gathered knowledge and gained experience in how to use many substances that help us heal energetically and find balance. This includes gemstones, crystals, minerals, food, herbs, oils made from plants and flower essences. All of these substances have specific energetic properties they offer to balance energies.

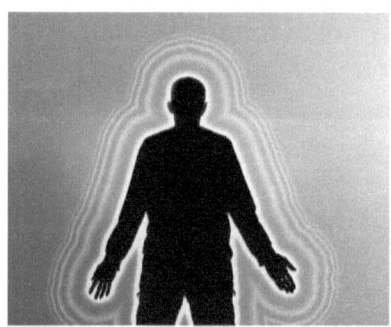

Humans are not just physical flesh and blood. Our mind/body/spirit complex is made up of layers of energy. Let's begin with the internal. Your very blood is pumping energy throughout your physical system, keeping your brain going and feeding all of your internal organs along with vast capillary beds hidden beneath your largest organ, your skin. Your blood moves through your entire circulatory and vascular system and is enhanced by the invisible life force energy which we can enhance through the practice of Qigong and Tai Chi. Whether you practice those body arts or not, energy is working in tandem with your blood to circulate the life force (chi) throughout your body system.

At the core of your body lies the incredible structure given to your physical form by your skeletal system. These are the bones you were born with that have grown over time. Additionally, they have the capacity, through the marrow, to make more stem cells for you which will then become red or white blood cells. It has been said that the energy internalized by the practice of Qigong is stored in the marrow of the bones to be called upon when needed for healing.

The muscular system that allows you to move those bones serves as a tremendous source of energy stored and exerted. Invisible energy also assists you in building muscle just as much as exercise and nutrition.

Your nervous system blends with your emotions. Whatever emotions you are feeling, your nervous system responds by triggering several events and sending signals and even hormones throughout your entire physical system. This is why it is very important to not ignore our feelings. Survivors must embrace all of their emotions, even the darker ones we find in our shadow side. By shining light and exposing these feelings, treating them with therapy and holistic practices, we heal them eventually and are able to attain better health.

Everything works together for a harmonious outcome or homeostasis. Here is a main difference between your genius physical body and the life force or chi. Your physical body ends at your skin. The reason you see it with human eyes, which are also a part of the physical, is because energy vibrates at a slower rate for physical manifestation. The slower the vibrating energy, the more solid the item appears. Qi mingles within your body and without. It is the invisible energy outside your physical body. Yet, it permeates your skin and other systems and comingles with your body to give it this vital life force energy. Just because we cannot see something, does not mean it does not exist. You cannot see radio waves, gamma rays and many other energy forms. Yet, they exist.

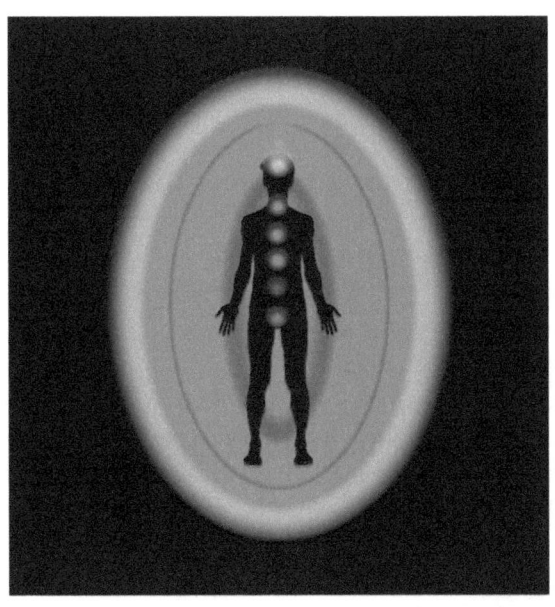

Chakra Energy Centers

Life force, energy or chi rotate within areas of our body via the seven primary chakras (pronounced chuhk-ruhs). Chakras are not seen by the human eye. However, their existence is spoken of now for thousands of years beginning in India. Chakras are like spinning wheels of energy in precise locations just outside the human physical body. They can be imagined as energetic portals or gateways because this is where the chi comingles with the human body. Chakras are encapsulated with the Subtle Body which is a field of energy made up of several layers including the etheric, emotional, causal, soul, lower mental and higher mental fields. It is not important right now to know all of what makes up the Subtle Body. Rather, it is beneficial to understand this is what exists outside of the human eye but has effect upon the entire body system. The term auric field is sometimes used for Subtle Body. Our Subtle Body contains all the information of everything that has happened to you in your life. The chakras reside in this first layer of the subtle body field. They join the physical body as each of the seven chakras corresponds to physical nerve ganglia which extend outward from the spinal column of each human.

When you experience blockages in one or more chakras, energy does not flow smoothly. This is the same principle we see with blood traveling through the veins. When veins or arteries become blocked, less blood is able to move through the vascular system at a given time. It is just as important to keep our chakras flowing in a steady manner. After all, we are talking about the energy of life force.

The opposite effect can happen when a chakra is too active or excitable. In this scenario, specific energy is causing almost a type of leaking of energy. Imagine a water valve left open a bit on accident. Interpret the water leakage that will occur as energy leakage from a chakra that is too open or over stimulated. When I speak of you losing or giving away your "power", this is what I am referring to. Your power or life force energy is dissipating in certain ways due to an imbalance in the emotional system or learned ways of living.

How do blockages and over activity occur in the chakras? There are many ways fueled by emotions and/or intense events. For sexual abuse survivors, it is common to carry part of that trauma within particular chakras. It is like an emotional imprint. Many sexual abuse survivors have traumas that can be trapped in these energetic portals. At times, an individual can have characteristics indicating that a chakra is too open and also blocked in some manner. In either case, bringing one's self back into balance is the goal and an attainable one.

In *The Magical Empath, Book I, Healing & Evolution*, I go into more detail about each chakra. For our purpose here, I will speak of particular challenges survivors may experience.

It would be a mistake to view the numbered chakras simply as levels of learning or accomplishment. You can be very clear minded, heart centered, well spoken and still have issues to balance in the first and second chakras. Imbalance can be cleared in the first and second chakras and later have different challenges that create imbalance. These chakras are not grades of learning where you begin at the first grade and advance to the second, third grade and so on. Numbers have only been assigned to the chakras for reference.

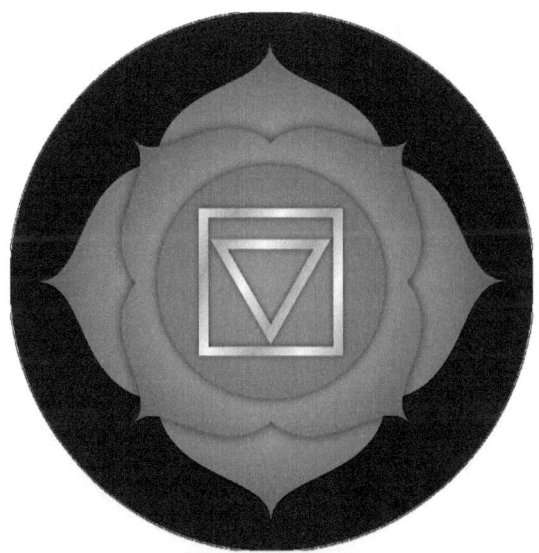

The Root Chakra

In Sanskrit, the first chakra is actually named Muladhara. Calling it by its original name may be better than the numeral system. It is important to realize that a person can be functioning in other chakras, yet have a need to balance a lower chakra. This does not mean you are a beginner. It just means something has shown up there that needs to be cleared so the entire system can flow more freely.

Muladhara means root support and it has often taken some hits with survivors of any type of trauma. This first chakra is your structure and roots that go deep into the ground of mother earth. In fact, the root chakra is ruled by the element of earth. One thing this chakra stands for is your physical body identity and, more so, your ability to meld with your body, knowing its needs and how to take care of it. We all have to be aware of what it takes for us to survive and thrive. The root chakra is very much about survival instincts and the will to live. It has much to do with our health and vitality. This is where chi enters into the body to help bring things into physical existence.

Located at the base of the spine, our root chakra governs how safe we feel in the world among other things. Trauma is easily stored in this chakra and this can cause blockages. Red is the color of the first chakra vibrational frequency. Conversely, you can have an excitability or over activity of this energy vortex.

A blockage could be felt as actual pain in the body at times including the lower back, coccyx area, thighs, knees, lower legs and feet. — areas under the influence of the root chakra. These would be physical manifestations. A blockage can make you experience fear and anxiety frequently. Other psychological conditions can include eating disorders and dissociation regarding personal identity. You also may surround yourself with clutter and dislike the task of organizing.

For those whose root chakra is too open or overactive, physical issues can include obesity and feeling sluggish with the amount of energy available upon exertion. Psychological or emotional manifestations of an overactive root chakra include hoarding; being resistant to change; and uncontrolled urges surrounding money.

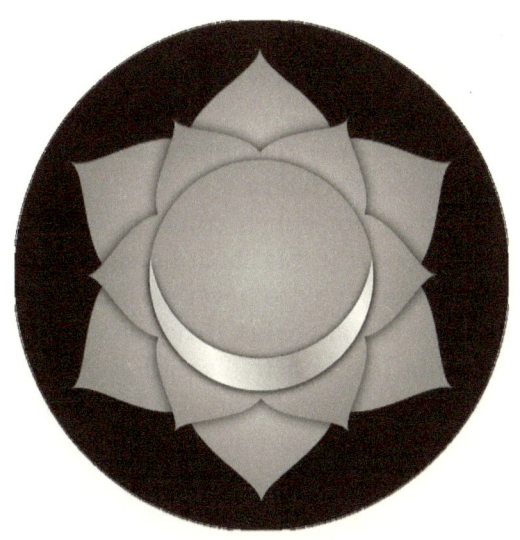

The Sacral Chakra

The second chakra is located a couple of inches below the naval and houses our creativity and sexuality. The element that rules this chakra is water which is much more mutable than earth. Water changes according to heat or cold. The emotions stored in this region do as well. In Sanskrit, the second or sacral chakra is named Svadhisthana which roughly translates to home of the self. This is where the watery emotions fuel creativity and sexuality. It is where we give birth to new selves literally or figuratively. Orange is the color vibration of this energy.

Due to the nature of your trauma, this chakra may easily experience blockages, be over stimulated or both. Much may revolve around impressions and judgments made about sexuality. On a physical level, blockage may eventually manifest as various diseases of the reproductive area or lower digestive issues. It can also manifest as sexual dysfunction such as the inability to attain arousal or orgasm. A blockage may leave one feeling as if they want to avoid pleasure when it comes to their sexuality. For some survivors, a blockage is indicated by the inability to feel — not just sexually, but their overall feelings. It is as if they are numbing themselves so they can avoid pain. If you suspect you may have excessive boundaries when it comes to interpersonal relationships, it could be from a blockage in the sacral chakra.

Certain behaviors which could be considered sexual addictions can occur if this chakra area is over stimulated. We also see those who are never sexually satisfied due to their overactive sacral chakra. Another clue that energy is leaking from an overly active sacral chakra is not having enough boundaries with others; promiscuity; feeling overly emotional; and having extreme ups and downs in mood.

The Power Chakra

The third chakra is located in the solar plexus region and its domain is the stomach, digestive system, liver, pancreas and gall bladder. It begins at the naval going up to just below the breastbone in the diaphragm area. Energetically, its color is yellow to gold and sometimes brown when really blocked. When this chakra is flowing well with energy, you feel free to express your ideas and exert your personal power in situations by stating preferences and making boundaries. When it is blocked, you may be very angry and blaming with other people around you. If this chakra is too open, you tend to lack boundaries and allow others to take advantage of you. Shame you may carry emotionally resides in this chakra area. It affects your projection into the world via your self-esteem.

The Sanskrit name of this chakra is Manipura and it corresponds with the element of fire. Manipura roughly means shining or lustrous gem. The power of your will is determined by the balance of this chakra. Have you heard the phrase, "the spirit is willing but the flesh is weak"? This exemplifies an out of balance situation where you may have the desire to do something, but lack the energy to carry through the task. When your third chakra is in an overexcited state, you may appear very controlling or competitive with others.

This area when balanced can improve your relationships with others in all facets of life and make you feel a true self-confidence. It will be easier to move forward with plans you wish to launch for your life.

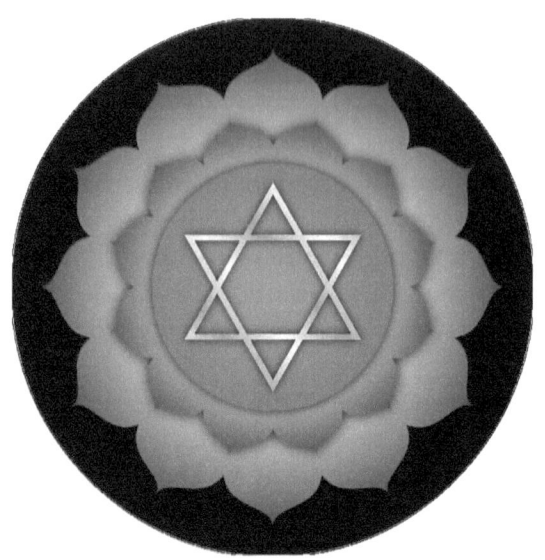

The Heart Chakra

The fourth chakra is known as the center chakra as there are three above it and three below it. This is the heart chakra and it rules not only the heart, but also the lungs and thymus area. The Sanskrit name for the heart chakra is Anahata which roughly means unhurt. Its element is air and the color is green. Here we find the emotions of unconditional love, joy and compassion hopefully stored. When this chakra is significantly blocked, it can be very difficult for us to love ourselves or others. We also may lack empathy for the pain or predicament of others. Physical blockages in this chakra can produce chest pain such as angina. Over time, it can manifest as actual heart, lung and breathing malfunctions. Emotional or psychological issues that show blockages within the heart chakra include feeling very alone; being critical of others; and not very sociable. When Anahata is too open, symptoms show up as being too giving — perhaps to the wrong people. Codependency is often present as well.

As a survivor, you may need to be reminded at times that you have the right to be loved. Receiving love is a fundamental right we are all born with. Due to the abuse, the idea that you deserve unconditional love for who you are may have disappeared. You may believe or feel that you have to earn love by doing certain things. You do not need to sacrifice yourself in any way, especially sexually, to earn love. You may find that you hold deep feelings that, unless you do things well, you do not deserve love. This belief may carry over into abundance factors of your life. As you unknowingly cut yourself off and say you do not deserve, you keep good from coming to you easily in many different forms. One of the ways that you can help heal blockages in the heart chakra is forgiveness of self. There is more information on self forgiveness in Chapter 20.

A practice that will help open and balance your heart chakra is a daily gratitude habit. There was a time a few years ago when certain thought leaders were encouraging people to state something each day of the year they were grateful for. This is a wonderful habit to develop as it assists in changing your focus on what is working and good. It is a key component to healing and balancing the fourth chakra. While a gratitude habit is an easy thing to implement, many people do not give their heart this gift because their focus is on what is lacking, instead of what is right there that they can love and be grateful for. Plus, it takes time to develop new habits. Challenge yourself to do this for one month and determine if it makes a difference for you. Ideas you could implement are writing down what you are grateful for each day in a journal or notebook. Alternatively, you could put it on small slips of paper and place them in a jar or some other container. When you are feeling down, pull one or two from the container and read to yourself.

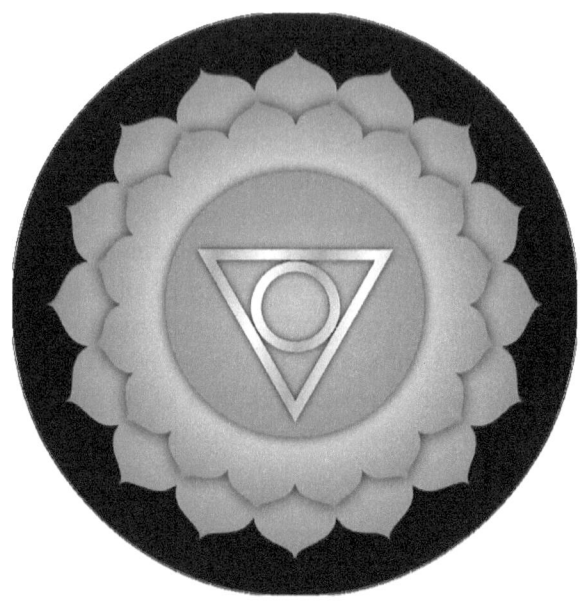

The Throat Chakra

The fifth chakra is located in the throat area and rules our ability to express ourselves and communicate our creative pursuits. Purification is what the Sanskrit name Vissudha means and this chakra with the element of sound has the capacity to soothe the body, mind and soul. Of course, sound is also vibrational energy. Our ability to speak our thoughts and desires resides here. The vibrational color is blue. In addition to the throat, the shoulders, thyroid gland, entire neck and jaw are affected by the throat chakra energy.

A common signal of blockage is experiencing frequent sore throats. As a child, this may have been recurrent if you were unable to speak of your abuse. Persons with blockages in the throat chakra may speak very softly to the point it is difficult to hear them. They may be afraid to speak for themselves or have a hard time putting spoken word to their thoughts.

An individual who speaks very loud or cannot stop interrupting others is a symptom of a throat chakra that is leaking energy. Have you ever been around someone who just cannot seem to stop talking and they go on about trivial things in an endless way? This would be another symptom of imbalance in the throat chakra.

This chakra is challenging for many sexual abuse survivors as they try to find a way to speak their truth or tell their story. It is imperative they tell someone and allow their secrets to be revealed to safe sources. Keeping this bottled up will certainly create imbalance in the throat chakra and affect them in many ways psychologically. If you have not done so already, consider downloading my free guided visualization which assists in revealing secrets such as the ones survivors hold.

Download at:
lyraadams.com

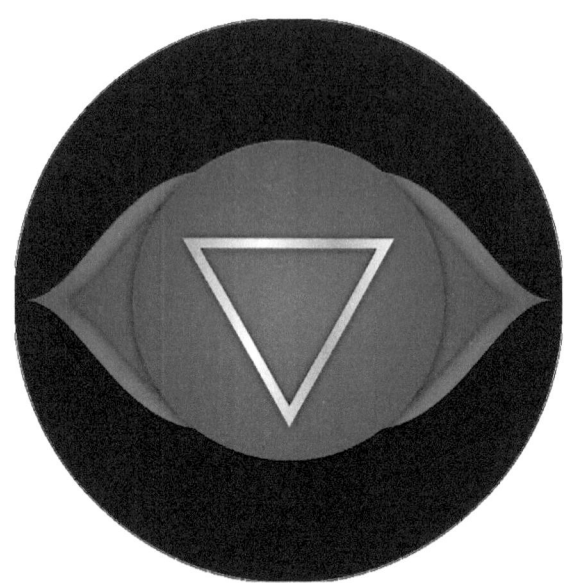

The Third Eye Chakra

Known as Ajna in Sanskrit language, this is the place of visions, dreams and intuitive knowing. Ajna roughly means to perceive and command and in this chakra area we find we are able to receive and put forth telepathically when it is operating well and balanced. It is located just above the eyes at brow level or a tad higher. Light is the element that rules the sixth chakra and its color is a deep indigo bordering on purple. Indications this area could be out of balance include headaches and dizziness where the area is experiencing blockage. If the imbalance is one of being overly open, hallucinations can occur. Nightmares may also be common.

For sexual abuse survivors, this chakra is prone to show us flashbacks or memories we may want to avoid. This could be triggered by outside events or even dreams. The third eye chakra is where many of these memories, but not all, are stored energetically in the subtle body. When a survivor avoids doing the work to heal the memories of the past abuse, the third eye can suffer from blockages. The longer this goes on, the more intense symptoms, both physical and psychological, can become.

The sixth chakra is where we do most of our "shadow work" as Jung called it. We go within during therapies to find the causes and learn to feel and grieve those happenings of the past. We do this by bringing them forth from the sixth chakra, then speaking them safely to the right people using our fifth throat chakra. Finally, we heal ourselves by grieving and finding compassion for our past and present person that we are via the heart chakra. This is a small example of how the energetic chakras interrelate with one another.

If you desire to be "clear seeing", identify imbalances that exist in this chakra and heal them.

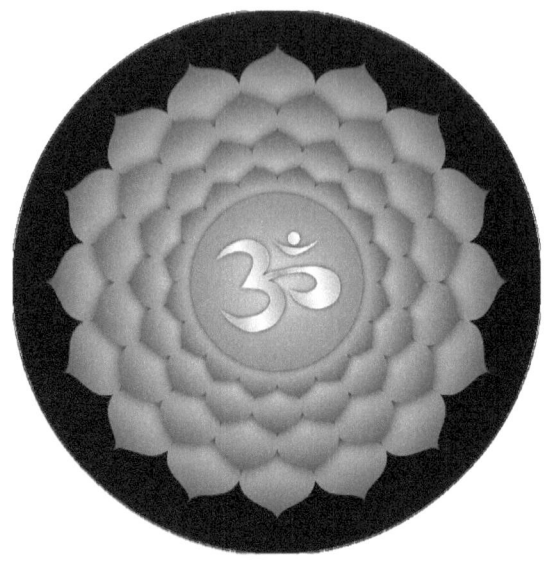

The Crown Chakra

Located at the top or just above our human heads, the Sanskrit name Sahasrara for the seventh chakra roughly means a thousand petals. When you have observed light filled halos around the head of individuals, this is the color vibration of the crown chakra. Within depictions for illustrations and paintings, the color of the crown chakra may be portrayed as white to gold and sometimes deep lavender or purple. Always, it is light filled.

Our seventh chakra allows us to commune with God Source or universal energy that created everything that is. It is where ideas come into our bodies. We then begin dreaming about how to make the idea a reality by using our intuition and perhaps even sleeping dreams. If we choose, we speak to the right people who may be able to assist us in making our idea into something tangible. Do you see how ideas are generated and flow downward through the chakra energetic system to become something in the physical once they reach the root chakra? We put our heart into the idea, followed by personal willpower to make it happen. Finally, we sprinkle it with creative love and perhaps some extra sauce to make it more marketable or appealing to others. Last, it comes into its fruition and rests fully formed.

Our seventh chakra allows us to tap into divine wisdom through the energetic threads of consciousness. This is where we can truly experience the oneness of everything. The energetic information relayed through this chakra is not tied to the limitations of earth and logical thinking. In fact, it produces a type of gnosis that is more of being an experiencer of the imparted knowledge than just a receiver of data.

Do you live in your head quite a bit of the time? Many survivors do this unknowingly. It is as if they feel more comfortable staying in the upper chakra region — hanging out there instead of coming down into the lower chakras where they may have to feel things. Symptoms you may be doing this in your life include being very left brain oriented. You want to think logically about things and not have too many feelings involved. While this is one way you unconsciously believe you are protecting yourself, the result is imbalance in the mind/body/spirit complex due to the other chakras being blocked with unhealed emotional trauma. When everything is flowing well from root chakra to crown chakra, we experience more joy and bliss. Our ideas that come to us from pure consciousness through the crown chakra are acted upon as we bring them into finality down to the root chakra. While invisible to our human eyes, it is a perfect system — a remarkable one that we are gifted with.

The chakras give us feedback on where we need to balance things emotionally. We can see this in symptoms we may carry at any given time. Our chakras, when listened and tended to, help us become balanced, healed and whole.

15 – Nature

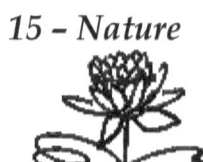

"One is nearer God's heart in a garden than anywhere else on earth" This is but one sentence from the poem *God's Garden* by Dorothy Frances Gurney. I remember glancing and reading those words repeatedly as a child in my grandmother's garden. Imprinted upon a metal plague that poked out of the ground in between lovely flowers, it was often the first thing that caught my eye. I would ask her, "What exactly does that mean? Is God here in the garden?" As I grew older, I discovered at moments that came upon me by surprise, the poet was right.

There is something otherworldly and magical about gardens, no matter how small. I came to view dirt, itself, as a substance that had a subtle power to not only feed plants which could eventually nourish our bodies, but as a method of absorption for our stress. It also works well with releasing anxiety, depression and other unwanted emotions. The discovery that putting my fingers in dirt made me feel better has kept me coming back again and again to feel it in my hands. I did not mind allowing it to ruin my painted manicure, the gift being higher than the cost.

Yet there is more to the euphoria produced from soil and plants in a garden. It's the gentle or strong breeze blowing across your face; sunshine beating down upon skin; or the smell of nature as it absorbs the nutrients from a recent rain. It could even be the wee folk or fairies hidden from human view as they sprinkle love and luck around. It is watching the insects as they participate in the great dance of life.

Now that you understand that your very being and everything around you is made of energy, seek environments that feed your spirit. This regular communion will allow you to feel lighter and happier. There will be days when you cannot do this. Of course, you may experience moments where it is hard to make yourself move from your chair or bed and get outside. Once you do, your energy will begin changing rapidly.

Being outdoors in nature is very healing for humans. Perhaps we were not meant to live inside four walls much of the time as we do. For all people, being outdoors around plants and animals can lift spirits greatly. That is why many people undertake gardening, working with plants in nurseries or florist shops.

Another beneficial therapy practice is working in the equine industry with horses. Many survivors of different types of trauma respond to animals better than people, at least for a portion of their lives. You may find them in a veterinary or animal grooming setting. Some work in animal shelters where cats and dogs have often been abandoned, neglected or abused. Of course, having a pet that is your companion is very therapeutic if you are in a position to do so.

The idea here is to get you out and about around plants, animals and nature. Do you live near the ocean? What an ideal landscape to enjoy and find solace. If you have a forest nearby that you could hike or simply enjoy sitting at a picnic table overlooking a lake or pond, this is ideal. Place your hands on a tree trunk. Lean into the tree, hug it if you want. Close your eyes and tell it your worries if you desire. The tree will absorb your lower thoughts you want to rid yourself of. Sit and journal at a park or botanical garden. Take some of your small crystals if you own them and hold them in your palms while lying in the grass.

Visit canyon or desert areas which contain a unique beauty of their own. In appropriate weather, open a window at night or sit on a porch and listen to the symphony produced by nature around you. Close your eyes and absorb it. Breathe and feel grateful as the earth envelopes you in joy.

Perhaps you could meet like-minded people who enjoy hiking, camping or rock climbing. Open your world and change your vibration by reconnecting with nature around you on a regular basis. This will speed your healing immensely.

Notes To Self

16 - Subtle Power of Flower Essences

It is amazing that something as fragile as the essence of a flower can have an effect on our energy and emotions. Flower essences work on the Subtle Body spoke of in Chapter 14. Many are very potent and a true gift from nature. Remember that we store many of our emotions in this auric body just outside our physical. Flower essences help us on an emotional energetic level.

Dr. Edward Bach (1886 - 1936) was an English physician who had a desire to discover how plants could help humans in a non-invasive way. He developed many combinations of flower essences he determined useful for balancing the emotions. Since he passed on to greater life, other flower essence practitioners have continued his research and therapy, working with adding new combinations.

Again, it must be remembered that our emotions stored are often creating imbalances for us in the way of blockage or being overly active in our physical body and auric field. When you are having difficulty even recognizing what makes you angry, sad, fearful, withdrawn, etc., the right flower essence can often make the difference as it soothes and brings balance.

Each flower essence is as different as the beautiful bud it emerged from. Just as each flower carries a unique scent, it contains an exclusive signature of its own that serves as a catalyst for healing particular emotional conditions. A flower essence used appropriately can help us release worn out patterns we have been stuck in for some time, gently eroding it away without pain.

The study of flower essence use is not taught in most academic settings. For someone wanting to become adept with the essences, it is helpful to work under a skilled practitioner and to study as many books as possible. Trial and error will be a teacher as well.

Many of us are aware and use herbal remedies for health and well being. They can be ingested a number of ways. However, flower essences are more delicate. Dr. Bach observed from being in nature and working with so many plants that the morning dew ingested had a very tonic and balancing effect on the human body. He hypothesized that the sun's energetic heat was encapsulating the properties of the flower into the dew droplets. It is not very convenient to try and find the right dew on the flower you need at just the exact time you need it. Dr. Bach developed a process he called sun potentizing. Still today, either Dr. Bach's sun potentizing or a boiling method is used to produce these fragile flower essences which help us on a vibratory level. There are many reputable suppliers around the world of flower essences. There are also many books with instructions on how to make your own. Ultimately, you will end up purchasing some because you may not have access to the particular flowers you need for holistic treatment.

Important Nutritional Factors

Your physical body and subtle body's health are connected. At times, you may have toxic situations going on that block vibrational remedies or energy medicine from working effectively. By eating healthy, taking supplements where needed, and avoiding alcohol and drugs, you will significantly assist your entire mind/body/complex in feeling its best. Plus, it will be more receptive to any type of vibrational healing.

Think about an individual who is alcoholic and drinks each day. How can a few drops of flower essence penetrate to their meridians and make their way into their subtle body for emotional healing? It's difficult. Yet, even too much caffeine or other substances can overload the central nervous system making it difficult to have proper functioning of vibrational remedies. This is also why the elimination of addiction is important. It will not only give you better overall health, it will clear mind/body/spirit complex allowing you to be more receptive to energy medicine of any type.

The healthier you are, the better flower essences work. Too much stress on the nervous system can serve as a blockage. Here are my recommendations for having the maximum benefit from your flower essences.

Keep stress low before use perhaps by lying down and listening to something relaxing. You can also use creative visualization or meditation to calm your mind/body/spirit complex. Holding a crystal such as black tourmaline may also assist you in returning to a neutral, yet grounded, state. Once you are calm, use your favorite method for ingestion of the flower essence.

In your daily life, make sure you are receiving enough nutrients — especially B vitamins which benefit the nervous system. Limit caffeine in coffee, tea and other sources that can over stimulate the central nervous system. Be aware that camphor can do the opposite by creating blockages in various sections of the auric field or subtle body. Camphor is more common than you might imagine. It is included in many cleaning products, cosmetics, muscle pain skin rubs, some bath salts and even as a food flavoring.

Other toxic conditions within the body that may block the receptivity of flower essences include aluminum and any other heavy metals from vaccines or the environment. If you believe your body may need a reset, consider a fasting period of three days where you ingest only pure fruit juices and water. You may also add fresh, watery fruits such as melons, berries and grapes for additional nutrition during the fast. Make sure to drink at least eight glasses of water during your fast. Overall, the cleaner you can keep your body temple, the better you will be able to absorb the life force from vibrational remedies such as flower essences.

If you are excited about trying flower essences, they are available from many different sources throughout the world. You can also find a selection of wildcrafted flower essences on my website – www. lyraadams.com

Use of Flower Essences

People use flower essences in numerous ways. The most direct way is to add 3 or 4 drops to a glass of water and drink. You can also use a dropper and place 3-4 droplets directly under your tongue. This sublingual fashion delivers faster results.

For prolonged, constant effects of a particular flower essence, consider adding 3-5 drops to a spray bottle filled with water. You may also add the same amount of drops to your favorite body lotion or cream. You will use more of the essence in a bath where it may take 15-20 droplets to have results.

Here are some very specific flower essences for survivors of sexual abuse trauma:

Religious or Ritual Abuse

For those subjected to abuse from religious leaders or ritual abuse of any sort, the flower essences of Loosestrife, Nectarine, Passion Flower and Queen Anne's lace are beneficial for balancing this particular emotional trauma. If you have anxiety or a fear of attending a temple, synagogue or church even for a wedding, try using Cotton flower essence.

Anger

Many survivors hold anger inside the very tissues of their bodies and the feathers of their soul. Anger always hurts us instead of the person we are angry with. Use the flower essences of Squash, Garlic or Centuary Agave to aid with unresolved anger.

Insomnia

Utilize the flower essences of Morning Glory, Chaparral or German Chamomile to aid with sleep. Sipping a cup of chamomile tea before bed can also help relax and prepare you for sleep along with a hot bath.

Dissociation or Identity Crisis

The flower essences of Four Leaf Clover, Bells of Ireland, Papaya, Mallow, Squash and American Paw Paw can assist you in healing issues making you feel as if you are splitting off or not knowing who you truly are.

Fears

For all fears, in general, use the flower essence of garlic. Note it will not have a garlic smell as this is from the garlic flower. That is a funny correlation between vampires and garlic, huh? Perhaps there is something to that. The flower essence of St. John's Wort is also a good selection for fears.

Self-Esteem

The beautiful flower essences of Iris, Jasmine and Daffodil are excellent to use for promoting greater feelings of love and appreciation for self.

Clearing Negative Thought Patterns

The flower essences of Comfrey, Forget Me Not, Orange and Live Forever are beneficial for helping to clear the subconscious mind. Also, the actual essence of Pine Tree sap is beneficial, but strong on smell.

Trauma

Star of Bethlehem flower essence is an excellent remedy for recent trauma. It is worth trying it for trauma of the past as well.

Shame and Guilt

The flower essences of Eucalyptus or Hyssop help to alleviate shame. With these two, hyssop is the stronger one. Eucalyptus helps us to grieve for that which hurts us.

Best Survivor Flower Essence

Overall, the supreme flower essence for trauma survivors is Lotus. When this is not available, you may substitute mango flower essence.

17 - Gems From The Earth

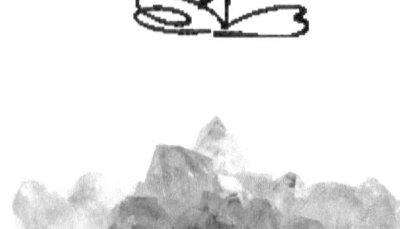

Did you ever pick up rocks or fossils you found as a child while exploring outside? Fascination with collecting any unusual rock I found began early for me. Once I discovered crystals, my entire world changed. In the beginning, I just felt they were beautiful. Later, I learned that each of them needed particular types of care and handling and were capable of giving off certain properties.

Over the years, I have been amazed at how well earth's gems can correct situations in our bodies and environment. The study of their ways of healing, restoring and balancing is years in the making. I hold respect for these incredible vibratory gemstones that will be here long after I leave. This is why precious gems are often given in the form of rings for marriage unions, representing something very long lasting.

Crystals are used to improve the living and working environments of many people around the world. They have the capacity to address vibratory states within the chakra system. Many are excellent tools for focus, creative visualization and meditation. Crystals have a long history of use around the world, supposedly as far back as the time of the fabled Atlantis and Lemuria.

All stones have some care requirements to keep them vibrating at their best energy. Some should never come in contact with water, while others are easily cleansed by it. Many are recharged in the sun, while others may require charging alongside other quartz crystals.

With loving care and respect, crystals have the power to brighten your world; heighten your intuition; calm your nerves; inspire your dreams; and focus your mind. There are numerous gemstones throughout our planet. Some are now rare and not found easily. This chapter will cover a few of the gemstones used for energy healing. I have chosen these gemstones, in particular, for abuse survivors.

Stones for Root Chakra and Grounding

Hematite

This is the perfect stone to calm your nerves and is very beneficial when feeling triggered. Hematite is actually a red stone, but often appears a combination of silvery black. The ground dust from hematite is red, probably from the iron oxide it contains. Its color makes it wonderful vibrationally for the root chakra area. If you are grieving or experiencing a difficult time, hematite can be a great companion as it strengthens you from within. Do not wear this stone on a regular basis. Use it for healing and grounding. It is too powerful to be worn all the time and could cause some inflammation in the body. Hematite should not be placed in water. Cleanse and discharge the energies picked up in this stone by placing it around quartz crystal.

Black Tourmaline

While we often gravitate toward beautiful sparkling crystals and stones, the solidity of black tourmaline can provide needed grounding for survivors of abuse. This stone also provides psychic protection to its owner. Black tourmaline correlates with the root chakra and is especially beneficial for those suffering from C-PTSD. You do not need a large stone for it to be effective. It can be rough or tumbled, but I prefer the rough stones when it comes to tourmaline as it shows the deep vertical ridges. Tourmaline actually has a magnetic charge when heated. Most pieces are primarily rectangular in shape and have a positive and negative at each end.

Another thing I like about black tourmaline is that I often take a moment to sit or lie down holding it when I am feeling overwhelmed. These feelings are usually brought about by too many things going on at once. After relaxing and holding my stone for just a few moments, I feel calmer and more focused to finish my tasks. This stone is excellent to hold when you are feeling emotionally out of sorts. Lying down, you may also place a piece of it at the first chakra to ground you into the earth. Some believe that tourmaline works by deflecting negative energy rather than absorbing it. To be on the safe side, cleanse this stone once a month under running water and place in the sun to recharge.

Obsidian

This stone is very prevalent and easy to obtain if you cannot find black tourmaline. It works similarly, yet is a little different. Expect to also feel more grounded while holding obsidian. This is a great stone when you are fearful or have anxiety from unknown causes. Discharge the energy it picks up every few weeks by running it under warm water and then placing it in the sun or among quartz crystals.

Clearing Stones

Pyrite

Have you ever seen Fool's Gold or Pyrite? You may have excitedly thought you came upon chunks of valuable gold, but this shiny mineral which resembles brass is not anything you can take to the bank. You can, however, use it to clear your body and living environment of negative energy — and that is pretty valuable. Pyrite will also absorb electromagnetic energy so it is great to keep around electronic devices that are emitting these vibrational frequencies. Some practitioners like to place a small piece of pyrite at the root chakra point and claim it increases energy significantly. Clean this stone by rolling it in salt. Do not let it come into contact with water. This stone loves the sun.

Smoky Quartz

While some use this hard quartz stone to ground their energy in the root chakra, it also clears your environment of negativity. By relaxing or meditating with smoky quartz, you may find it calms your emotions. This is another gem that assists in mitigating electromagnetic radiation in your environment. Take care of smoky quartz by discharging the energies it picks up once per month. Do this by placing it under running water and charge it by placing upon or among quartz crystals.

Azurite

Azurite is very good for cleansing the subconscious — we all know that we have things buried there. This stone is associated with the third eye and crown chakras. It should be cleansed of energies it picks up about once a month by placing it among hematite stones. Azurite contains powerful energy and does not need to be recharged.

Topaz

This is a gorgeous yellow gem that has been used in healing for centuries. Topaz is detoxifying to the system, especially some of the internal organs associated with the third chakra. It calms the nervous system and inspires creativity within the user of this stone. Topaz should be cleaned after each use by running under water. Recharge in the sun.

Balancing Stones

Tiger's Eye

This beautiful stone is sometimes called cat's eye. It correlates primarily with the third or solar plexus chakra. Tiger's Eye can assist you in bringing your entire mind/body/spirit/complex into alignment and balance. It can assist in lifting you out of depression. Discharge this gem under running water and recharge in the sun. Only wear Tiger's Eye for a few days at a time. Otherwise, it could interrupt the flow of chi.

Rutilated Quartz

If you feel depressed or are just in a bad mood, this species of quartz crystal assists in clearing and balancing your emotions. Beyond that, it is a powerful stone that can assist in clearing any blockages you have in the chakras. As it clears these embedded wounds that are blocking an area, it uplifts your spirits greatly. Cleanse this stone once a month under running water and place in the sun or among quartz crystals to recharge.

Amethyst

Amethyst is an ideal crystal to use in conjunction with rose quartz as it brings a beautiful balance of mental and emotional energies. Amethyst helps the mind as rose quartz helps the heart. Amethyst is traditionally linked to third eye usage and is protective and purifying to your entire mind/body/spirit complex. Consider placing amethyst clusters in areas where you work or live as they assist in ridding your environment of negativity. Amethyst does not like to be placed in the sun. To cleanse, place it under running water and among hematite to recharge.

Jade

For balancing emotional stress or if you are experiencing aggravated symptoms of C-PTSD, Jade is a great stone to turn to. Many survivors are empathic and highly sensitive. This can bring about a great deal of anxiety at times. Use this stone to wash away those feelings. Jade aligns with the third and sixth chakras. Cleanse it periodically under running water and place it on an amethyst cluster to recharge.

Carnelian

This stone is usually orange in color but may contain some yellow or red as well. Often, there are small spots or inclusions of brown. Wear this stone if you are battling depression so that it is making direct contact with your skin. For those that carry this stone, it gives added energy. Cleanse it once per month under running water and allow it to recharge for a couple of days in the sun.

Sugilite

When you have to endure hard memories from the past, this stone can be a true friend. Sugilite calms your nervous system and bring you back into balance and control. Discharge it once per month by placing it around hematite. This stone carries so much energy it does not need a recharging period.

Chrysocolla

If you fly off easily into anger, this stone is perfect to wear or have in your pocket. Feelings of hate dissipate with Chrysocolla. This stone calms and makes one more tolerant of situations, building their intuition to point them towards resolution of situations rather than "war". Clean once per month under running water and allow the stone to recharge near hematite.

Love Stones

Self-love is almost always lacking in abuse survivors. From deeply questioning their personal value to feeling safe enough to be loved, the right gems can assist greatly.

Rose Quartz

If there is one stone I feel correlates well with our inner child, it is rose quartz. This is a perfect stone to wear or carry in your pocket. It specifically targets the fourth heart chakra area. It's very much a stone that soothes the emotions. It is calming and makes you feel better about yourself. For those who need to develop more self love, rose quartz is a perfect stone to wear and keep around you. It would not hurt to keep rose quartz in rooms where you spend a great deal of time whether that is an office, kitchen or bedroom. It helps heal internalized pain and emotions trapped in the heart. I do not recommend that you wear a pendant that is too close to the heart. Perhaps, wearing it at the neckline or as a bracelet would be better. The reason is that the closer this stone is to the heart, the more it could activate your emotions as you cleanse the heart chakra area. Rose quartz needs to be cleansed often of the negativity it absorbs. Run it under water about once a week and recharge it by placing it near or upon an amethyst cluster.

Kunzite

This beautiful pink and lavender stone may be used with rose quartz for a boosted effect. It specifically helps those feeling inner turmoil and promotes feelings of self worth and love. It can be helpful for the treatment of addictions as well. Kunzite helps you build inner fortitude and tolerance. The pink in the stone correlates with the heart chakra and the purple with the sixth chakra. When using Kunzite, wear it so that it is touching your skin. This stone must be cleansed after each use by running under water. Recharge it by placing it around hematite.

Citrine

This yellow to gold colored crystal rules the third chakra area. It is helpful for stress, depression and nervousness. It assists in building self confidence and giving renewed enthusiasm. It works best if it is making skin contact with you. Unlike many crystals, this one should be cleaned after each use by running under water. Recharge it in the sun.

Notes To Self

18 – Sound

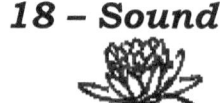

The right sound has the capacity to immediately improve your mood. Used regularly, it may change your entire outlook on life going forward. Used holistically, the methods spoken of here in this chapter are ancient, yet growing as a healing modality. In fact, many are being used today. Healing techniques with sound may be used by anyone, not just survivors of sexual abuse.

As you are probably aware but perhaps do not always think of it, sound is a vibration. You are now aware that all of life is made of energy. Everything in our world – absolutely each thing you can see, smell, touch, hear or sense is made of energy. Even the molecules that comprise a rock are vibrating at a particular frequency that gives the mineral its composition, feel and appearance.

Energy is made up of sub-atomic particles that are vibrating at different rates of speed. This speed is also known as frequency. The atoms in the very object you are sitting, standing or lying upon right now are vibrating. While we cannot see or feel this, if looked at through an electron microscope, moving particles can be detected. Amazingly, you are also vibrating at a certain frequency.

Sound vibrations are measured as a frequency that is traveling toward us in wave like patterns. It can exist at different rates of speed. There are some sounds you may not be able to hear with your human ears because they are below or above the frequency you pick up. Often, animals can pick up on sound vibrations we cannot. Even though you may not be able to hear those frequencies, they still exist and can have an effect on you.

When we have sound waves coming toward us, a process goes on that adjusts our own body and mind's resonance to those sounds. This is why you feel more relaxed and at peace when you hear ocean waves, the sound of crickets on a summer evening, or light classical music. Likewise, it is what gets your blood pumping, speeding up your heart rate with excitement when you hear music such as rock, heavy metal, rap and other more common selections today.

Ancient healers knew that specific sounds could provoke states of deep relaxation. Shamans often use sound to induce trance states. The right sounds can accelerate emotional healing from trauma of any type. As our mood changes with the sound and we experience the change, sound can assist us in releasing loneliness, depression, anxiety and fears. While these beautiful calming sounds can help us emotionally, they also work on our physical bodies which are made up mostly of water. The liquid in our bodies receives those healing sound vibrations, helping us to address aches, pains, muscular problems and serious chronic disease. Sound therapy has also been shown to be useful for those undergoing healing from surgery, and even those ready to pass on who are receiving hospice care.

As stated earlier, everything – absolutely everything is made up of energy that is vibrating at different rates of speed. These vibrations produce a resonance. During the 1600's, a Danish scientist found that two pendulum clocks placed side by side would eventually synchronize. The amazing thing is that this also happens within our own body system as we attune with the harmony and rhythms in our atmosphere. This is known as entrainment. Deep changes can be made in the brain with nothing more than sound. I think that is truly remarkable for those wanting to heal from trauma. Sound can actually help us at a brain level. Feelings and thoughts you carry in your mind are affected by how you are resonating. Therefore, if you listen to sounds that are more positive and healing in vibration, your mind and body system will begin to match those sounds in resonance through this process called entrainment. While this sounds like magic, it is actually just physics.

Sound and light can be imagined as coming into existence via waves – waves of energy. These waves are measured in hertz. Many believe that the rate of all healing music can be measured in hertz which reduce numerically to 3, 6 or 9. Coincidently, these are the same principal numbers Tesla wrote of, saying they were the keys to the universe. This system is known as the Solfeggio frequencies.

Here is an example of how to reduce the hertz music is flowing at down to one numeral:

If you are listening to sound projecting at 432 Hz – simply take 4+3+2. This equals 9.

Let's say it is 528 Hz – take 5 + 2 + 8 equals 15, but since you have two numbers there, add them together. 1+5 equals 6. To know if the sound fits into the healing hertz range, it should always be 3 or a single numeral divisible by 3. This correlates with the Solfeggio frequencies.

There are some purists who insist that only 432 Hz is beneficial, relating it to the Schumann resonance, a set of electromagnetic oscillations that originate from earth. I have personally found that all music which reduces to a 3, 6 or 9 feels beneficial to me. It might be a fun experiment for you to try different selections to see how or if you are affected emotionally or physically.

While this is really conjecture about the different Hz, it is possible that all music at any Hz can have an effect upon us. I tend to believe this is so. However, I also know that certain sounds are more calming and definitely feel more healing. Many of those sounds come from nature such as the sound of water falling upon rock. The symphony of frogs and crickets in the forest at night can lull you toward sleep. Certainly, the gentle waves and more robust ocean sounds calm our spirit.

Did you know that color is a vibration? Color is refracted light and it also corresponds to musical scales. This suggests there is a correlating factor between sound and light vibrations. I know of some musicians who have had regular, but unpredictable, instances of seeing color in their mind while playing their instrument.

In my studies and practice of balancing the human energy body, I have learned it also is affected by incoming waves of vibration like sound and light. Each of the seven energy centers of the body, or chakras, correspond to the same primary colors of the musical scale, beginning at red at the first base chakra and ending in violet at the seventh crown chakra. The color violet has the shortest wave when measured.

Solfeggio Frequency Characteristics
396 Hz — Releases Fear
417 Hz — Eases and Initiates Change
528 Hz — Healing and DNA Repair
639 Hz — Heals Relationships
741 Hz — Finding Creative Expression and Solutions
852 Hz — Spiritual Homecoming

These frequencies can expand your thinking, give clarity, promote healing on emotional and physical levels, and make you feel better ... perhaps an intense love state at times. They can lower blood pressure and have amazing effects on the organs of the body. Your feelings really matter. The way you feel emotionally is dictating a lot of what goes on in your body, mind and life.

Try changing some of the music you listen to. Ever notice how many songs speak of lovers done wrong and victimhood? It is so pervasive and much has been said about people wanting to wallow in their misery. Yet, realize you are programming your mind each time you engage in this. There is something to be said of sorrow, grief and loss, but we don't want to stay there in it. What if you listened to things that evoked different feelings in you?

One of the things I really love about sound healing is that you can play some music while you are engaged in other activities. Whether you are walking your dog in a park, doing your laundry or washing dishes, you can listen through ear buds or in the background at home through another device. It is a very simple way to change how you are feeling. The more you do it, the greater the effect will be.

There are many forms of this music available for download or listening online. You want to search for particular frequencies and perhaps try out a few of them to see how they change how you are feeling. It might be a good idea to keep a notebook of which ones produced different moods. Some may make you feel very tired and sleepy. Keep this in mind as I do not recommend listening while driving or doing any task where being very alert is important.

The human voice is also an instrument. It can be used to soothe, heal, excite or invoke many different emotions. Chanting, singing and even speech can be forms of therapy. There will be some voices you do not care for. For whatever reason, the voice may bother you in some way.

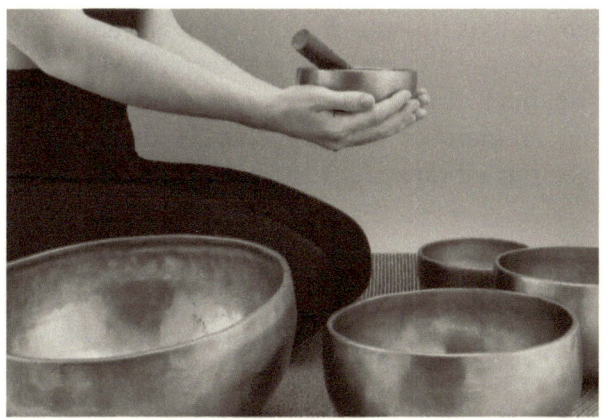

Have you ever heard Gregorian monk or Tibetan monk chants? Many people find those vocal compilations healing. The ancient sound of drumming is wonderful for working on first chakra issues. Tibetan singing bowls produce wonderful sounds that resonate so well. You can find them made of metal and quartz. The bowls come in sets of seven, although you may purchase each individually as well. Each bowl produces a different frequency that correlates with a particular chakra or note on the scale. You can also use tuning forks for assisting in the balance of the chakras.

Something to be aware of while you experiment with listening to different frequencies of music is this: once you begin to notice how the sound vibrations make you feel different inside, people, places and things that surround you on the outside may begin to feel more annoying or difficult than usual. This is a very natural reaction because you are changing your vibrational state and you are noticing what is not matching up with you. Just be patient with yourself and others at this point. Be aware, however, that it this feeling of incongruence or not matching up could be showing you what needs to change in your outer world. We can never change others, but we can change our responses to things around us. We can decide if it is something that fits into the life we want and, if not, what changes we need to make on a personal level.

The next time you are experiencing any negative feelings, remember to play sounds that will help you change your vibration.

Notes To Self

19 - Mental Focus

You were born a unique, whole being -- one full of tremendous potential and possibilities. Some hear that message and very much own it. Some hear those words and, while they understand it on an intellectual level, have a difficult time really feeling it. And there are valid reasons to struggle with truly owning the concept.

First, is the concept of personal power. What is personal power? It is not exerting mental or physical force upon yourself or another. To stand in your own power means you feel comfortable being you and letting others around you know where you begin and they end. It means you do things because you want to instead of out of fear of not being loved, appreciated, or included in some way. Personal power means you take responsibility for your experiences in life.

Most humans have experienced being a victim of something or someone. These happenings often leave deep grooves in our psyche. Removal can seem daunting at times. Yet, in order to transform from victim to victor, we must take active responsibility in our circumstances.

One of the first concepts I learned in my healing studies centered on responsibility. Responsibility, as I was taught, means my ability to respond and how I choose to do that. It is the way I choose to react to situations or how I frame things that have happened. I have the power to choose. For your new life ahead, remember that you are responsible for how you feel, not others. You always have the power of choosing how you will respond.

Part of being a victim is feeling out of control. Many survivors have issues that pop up regularly around the concept of control. We also have patterns we are trying to eliminate. Things that are extremely difficult, but others may not even see. We often feel like life is not really working for us or the way we want it to.

Often, we live our lives feeling like there are two parts of us engaged in a tug of war. There is the part of us that wants to create great new experiences and achieve things we know we deserve but have not yet had come into our life. Then, there is the other part that seems to be working against this – the part that says we do not deserve. This battle is going on inside many people – not just sexual abuse survivors. Most of the people on this planet walk around each day not feeling good enough. And they keep repeating patterns that indicate that is what side of the war is winning.

In order to change this and allow in a better new life and the experiences that go along with it, we have to change our focus. We have to start telling that part of us which I often refer to as the negative ego to shut up. Tell it to take a vacation. Let that part of you be the losing team. It's part of the old story – not the new one you are creating.

Instead, begin focusing on what is going well in your life right now. If you look closely, you will see that there are many things working in your favor. If you are still feeling quite traumatized by the events that happened, this can be extremely difficult. Regardless of how long it has been, let's start with things that are basic to change focus. Because when we change the way we think, things around us begin to change. We make more headway on our healing journey in a faster and deeper way.

Depending upon the type of trauma inflicted, this can be difficult to take notice of. But, this is where I would like you to start. I always suggest that people begin with what feels easy. New ideas may be added as you ramp up your healing recovery. Start out with easy and then move forward. This is one of the ways we can begin to feel victorious, instead of controlled by the dynamics of something that happened prior.

Trauma healing takes a lot of time. There are little gifts along the way in which you make tremendous head way in a short time. For the most part, however, you need to be patient with yourself. Often, it can begin as a change in how and what you are focusing on. So, let's explore that. What could you begin with that you know you can believe? Let's start with your physical body.

Right now, there are thousands of processes going on to keep your physical body in homeostasis. You are not aware of them. You don't even think about them. This is all happening inside of you but you are not really conscious of it. Can you see how there is something greater than yourself taking care of you all the time? Although you may be ill, injured or paralyzed, think of the parts that are still working correctly. If you have cancer in one or two parts of your body, reflect on the millions of healthy cells that make up every area of your body except those one or two. What a miraculous thing the human body is. On auto-pilot, it is constantly guided to heal and find homeostasis. Even our brains work to try and protect us, by allowing us to slip into denial when events are too overwhelming. This protective measure should be temporary, of course, but it is just another example of how our body is taking care of us all the time in the best way it can.

Have you ever thought deeply about an element like water? Water gives life and is essential to it. Water can become so extreme and powerful that it can take life. Yet always, if you tried to pick this liquid up in your hand, some would slip through your fingers. Water is so soft, yet the constant movement of it can carve rock. Water can become hard when exposed to the right temperature. Likewise, it can evaporate right before your eyes when exposed to enough heat. You cannot be water but water is a good portion of what forms your body. It is beyond a chemical. It is a compound element that forms the basis of life. How miraculous is that? Who or what makes water happen? Think deeply on this to feel the depth of miracles in your environment and in yourself.

What if you just decided to go through an entire day feeling lucky? Try navigating with the thought "I always have good luck. Everything I need comes to me easily because I am so lucky." Repeat that affirmation to yourself over and over. If you do this, first you will notice that your feelings begin to change. Putting emotion behind it makes this happen. If you're driving to work, yell out "I am so lucky!" If you hit a traffic jam due to a wreck ahead, say to yourself "I am so lucky that I am here and not in that wreck." By deciding how you will respond, you can turn many situations into your good fortune. It does not have to be something where you are more focused on being late. Maybe you are lucky to be late. Perhaps you avoided something by being where you are. You are lucky – think it – say it with emotion – feel it and you will find yourself in a lucky mood all day.

These simple ways of being responsible and rethinking things are the beginning of the new, better you. By changing the way you are responding to your life, you begin to silence the victim mode and reach toward something greater that is already inside you, just buried and in need of retrieval. You were born for your own greatness and it is there. Begin anew each day and practice positive things like this over and over. Through rote and repetition, you will become so different than you were before. You will begin to heal that part of you that has been retaining its hurt for too long.

During this time of reinventing yourself, fill your mind with healthier thoughts and feelings fueled by intense emotion. Give up that which is not serving you. Walk away from watching negative things on television that are not propelling you forward to the new you. Fill your time with thoughts of the future – hopefully very near future. Look up places you would love to travel to. If possible, collect photos of these places and start a vision board for your new adventures.

Imagine people in your new life who are supportive, loving and healthy in their responses to you. Daydream about this each day and you will attract those people to you at the perfect, right time. Affirm "I attract people to me that are loving, healthy and supportive of each other."

See yourself handling your finances with a new finesse you did not have before. Deftly take care of balancing accounts and keeping track of things responsibly and with care. You save money for yourself and invest in things wisely. You give appropriate sums of money away with forethought and without needing anything in return.

What do you fantasize about that you have not accomplished? Make a bucket list of items you want to do for the next few years. See yourself doing them.

Daydream and see yourself fully functional with opportunities constantly for you to grow. See yourself ready more than ever to handle whatever situation you find yourself in. Envision being surrounded by relationships and people who are understanding and loving. Light an inner fire to recite affirmations you can believe in. Trust that even if you hear doubts arise in the beginning, these are just memory reflections stored in your subconscious and they will finally subside and go into a long sleep or disappear entirely.

With what you have endured in the past, you have already walked through the fire. You may have danced through it. That story is a part of you, but it is not the totality of you. You are so much more! You have uncovered a good portion of it, but sometimes you must go deeper into the pond, into the darkness and examine it again to see how it may be affecting you. How can you help others if you do not perform the rescue upon yourself? Especially if at a core level you feel not good enough or flawed in some way. You do this by exploring where you hold onto the negative and notice when you are thinking that way in your mind. Trauma, neglect, abandonment issues are often found at the bottom of this. As you shine light on these shadow issues you have been carrying deep within, healing begins to occur.

How do you get through this maze of negative emotions and live your new life? It is through personal analysis combined with new habits and retraining of the mind. We have the capacity to burn away that which plagues us. We always have the choice to take the higher road in circumstances. We are on a personal growth journey toward our best selves and the only way this can happen is by encountering some adversity and meeting it head on where and when we can.

Everything we explore in our life has purpose. We are advancing our tools for dealing with our past, even when it was as recent as yesterday. As we heal, we transform our lives. When we truly understand that the more we change internally and do the work, we see things change externally. When we heal ourselves, we truly help heal the world.

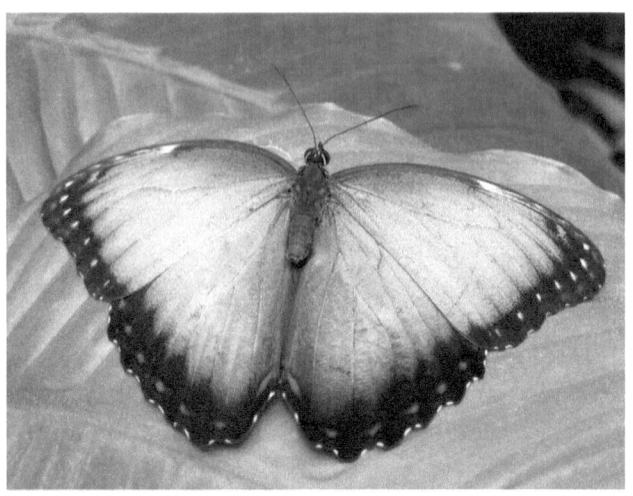

Signs of Transformation

One day, you awake and find you are not who you were a year ago. Because of all the recovery work you have accomplished, you know that you are not now who you will be in the near future. Your petals are unfolding, gently and beautifully to greet the sun. Yet, the transformation process is still in motion. You are in an emerging state from the muddy pond — opening to life and all the possibilities it holds for you.

You have experienced deep healing that has transformed you on a cellular level. Once again, you feel free to examine your feelings and are not afraid to allow every emotion to wash over you. In awe, you look back at how far you have come. Yet, you know old ways will pop up and reveal things you still need to clear — feelings keeping you in the fight-flight-freeze mode.

Overall now, trauma from the past is not dictating your present or future. As old patterns appear, you utilize your well earned knowledge to clear them. As their grip is loosened, you watch yet another petal open and kiss the sun. You are becoming more content, comfortable in your skin and wise.

Creative Visualization

Einstein once said that "imagination is more important than knowledge". And, it is. Imagine artificial intelligence with vast knowledge, but no imagination. While knowledge is important, using our minds to daydream and create artificial circumstances can prove very fruitful.

The process of creatively visualizing a scenario you would love to see unfold can actually help it come into your world. This is not fantasy. It is real because everything works on vibration, remember? Everything begins with a thought first. In other words, it must be imagined into existence.

Before you purchase a house, you must imagine that you want one. You might daydream about the location and features of your future home. At some point, you either receive the money for such an investment or obtain a loan to make it a reality.

Everything you want in life begins with a thought. Spend time visualizing what you desire.

Affirmations, Prayer and Meditation

The power of affirmations, prayer and meditation is a threefold combination that will absolutely propel you forward in your life. Each is different and provides unique results.

Affirmations are an excellent way to retrain the way you think. Throughout this reading, there has been mention of how our negative ego says very harsh, nasty things to us at times. This subconscious part of us battles at times with our rational mind. We know what it is saying is not true, but still it can win out. By repeating affirmations to yourself on a regular basis, you will begin retraining your negative ego. Now, it will learn wonderful things instead of negative messages you picked up along the way from many sources.

If you believe in a higher power, allow yourself to commune with that God Creator in prayer. Prayer is when you speak to God and lay your burdens on the Great Creator's altar to be dealt with in ways you cannot currently comprehend. When you don't know how to find a solution or just need to cry and ask why, this is the time to go to God in prayer.

Meditation is a beautiful practice where you quiet your mind and just listen. This is your opportunity to possibly hear God's answer. While meditation does not come easily to most people, it is often made more difficult by trying too hard. Relaxation with your breath is key. As you practice it more, you will soon be able to focus on nothingness. It is within this nothingness that peace can be achieved and answers or ideas are often received.

Choose one or all three of these methods for lighting a fire under your recovery. All are holistic practices that are beneficial to you. Your brain has the ability to rewrite its programming by engaging in practices such as meditation, affirmations and prayer. You will actually create more neural pathways in your brain as you allow in healthy feelings and thoughts.

Notes To Self

20 - Self Forgiveness

You never have to forgive those who have abused you. Your healing will progress without doing so. However, you may hit a certain point in your recovery where some type of forgiveness happens toward your perpetrators. This is different for each survivor. Every story and effect is unique. Realize you do not have to feel true forgiveness for those who hurt you. You may honestly not be able to. But, you can still heal.

The important thing you must do is forgive yourself. Too often, we hold ourselves hostage in life because we are running a very quiet background program inside that says we could have prevented something from happening. It is also common to hold contempt for ourselves for wrong choices we make after the fact. Forgive yourself for this as well. Realize that you are only capable of operating and conducting your life with the tools and knowledge you have present at any given moment. Additionally, many sexual abuse survivors carry a type of programming that went on during their abuse that makes them "act out" their abuse in strange ways after the fact. This can happen in a number of ways. It shows up in our lives as choosing the wrong people to hook up with; being attracted to certain places, people or things that somehow have a distant or close connection to our original abuse. Forgive yourself for this. You are healing and deprogramming. Now, you would not make those same decisions. Now, you know different. However, you are blaming yourself for past choices. Let it go. Moving forward, you must be free of the self-contempt that originates from this blaming of self.

I understand the blaming of self and reached a point where I knew I needed a clean slate to work with. There is emotional pain as we look at the darker things that happened to us. One of the darkest aspects I had to face were the things I did on my own – ways I acted and people I engaged with after the abuse.

It is not uncommon to be promiscuous after sexual abuse. In fact, it is very common. As you mature, you may hold shame about that also. If you are still engaging in it, you may carry a combination of denial such as thinking I don't care and a layer of shame at the bottom that you do not always see. However, on a certain level, you feel this shame. I am not telling you that I think you should feel ashamed for anything you do. However, if you do feel it, it needs to be addressed. As long as it is there, you will not feel comfortable in your skin.

Another common thing survivors experience is that they unconsciously engage in relationships with others who are on some level like their prior abusers. Addictions are often acquired by people who have been abused because they assist in avoiding our feelings. Because you know your addiction is not good and society reiterates that to you, this creates more shame and possible self loathing that you carry.

There are two ways to look at what you loathe about yourself:

The first: everything that happened to you and anything you did in response to it after the events is over. It is not what is happening now as you are trying to heal yourself. In fact, you have bravely swum through strong currents to get to where you are now. You are a survivor and are no longer being victimized in that way. Try to bring yourself into the mindfulness concept of the "now" each time you feel conflict about yourself. Regain control over what you are focused upon. For instance, at any given time, we are either living in the past, present or future. By being in the present, we greatly improve our ability to cope with whatever is around us.

The second is forgiveness. You must forgive yourself for everything you have participated in. With forgiving yourself – do not fret over things you did or did not do after your abuse. This correlates with staying in the now and not looking back. If you knew the statistics and how common it is for people to act out in strange destructive ways after being abused, you would feel like you had so much company in the world. So, give yourself a break dear one. Let it go – cry if you want – journal about it if you choose to – but then let it be over. The person you are right now today has grown and is continuing on that path. Forgiveness of yourself is such an important part for you to be able to forge ahead. When we forgive ourselves, it means we can now move forward into the future. We can be in present moment knowing that we did the best we could under the circumstances and move into the future with a clear conscience knowing that not only have we forgiven ourselves, but we have poured compassion upon our hearts. If you are a Christian, your religion teaches you to ask God for forgiveness. That may be done as well. It is important, however, for you not to carry guilt — to forgive yourself for whatever you feel your participation or lack thereof was in any situation. It may be hard at first to forgive yourself. Remember, you do not need at any point to forgive those who hurt you. You can if you wish and you truly feel that. Forgiveness for the way you have been transgressed by others may take time. It may never happen. That is okay as well.

Each time you begin to worry about what other people would think if they knew what you had done or things you did not do, STOP! If people really love you, they try to understand you – all of you – not just the parts you want to present to them. That is truly honoring and loving someone. Plus, you do not have to reveal all your secrets to everyone. In fact, I would only do so with those that really count in your life. Understand that in your own way, you have always been trying to cope and do your best.

It is important to take time to grieve for the child, teen or adult that was traumatized by abuse. This grief can be stimulated through the act of actually crying. Whether you sob lightly or more intensely, crying and feeling the grief is good to help you enact self-forgiveness. It may be wise to have a very good friend with you when you engage in the grieving process as many feelings can come up possibly triggering challenging responses from you. As you release the deep feelings via crying, your heart opens and you become lighter. These tears of compassion you are pouring upon yourself are heartfelt and you richly deserve this empathy.

My hope is that your healing will be spectacular and that you will finally feel so comfortable with who you are. You will no longer feel any self-hatred, shame, or loathing. Instead, you will be a champion for each aspect of yourself – your inner child and the adult you are now. It is all possible and I believe in you. You will look back upon the journey you walked and be proud. Do the work – that's key – reach out for help when you need it – that is important too. With forgiving of self, you open more petals to fully bloom.

At times, it is easy to feel angry that we have to spend so much time trying to heal or fix ourselves. Yet, there are golden gems discovered about you and life along this healing journey. Discovery often happens when you are not expecting it and the more you heal, the more frequent these gifts of insight occur. They allow you to build self worth and confidence. Ultimately, you are bringing peace of mind into your world.

Holistic Helpers

I came across the recommendation of a rare crystal called Linarite. While I have never worked with this gem, it is said to assist with releasing negative emotions and feelings we have buried deep inside. It also works on the fifth chakra area (throat) allowing us to speak our true feelings more easily.

Malachite is a stone I want to highly recommend for many purposes. For self forgiveness, this gorgeous green gem works on the fourth heart chakra area. It has the ability to show us what lurks in our subconscious and needs clearing. As this inner debris begins to come to the top of the muddy pond, we can clear it by placing malachite in the solar plexus or third chakra area where many repressed emotions are stored. Additionally, by adding a clear quartz crystal, this will give you added benefits. Be aware that because malachite works in the way it does, it is not a stone to wear on a frequent basis. Rather, this stone with its myriad of purposes is best used during relaxation, visualization or meditation.

Notes to Self

21 - Self Love

Love -- we all want it, but many of us wonder if we will find the right kind of love. Some of us still wonder what love really is. Others are not sure they are worthy of love. Unfortunately, this can easily happen with people who have been abused.

I would like to share with you something I learned about love – we must give it to ourselves first. And, it cannot be fake love. It has to be a real love we feel inside that overrides all the negative programming we have picked up so far. How do we do it -- especially after enduring so much hurt from others? It requires courage and being brave enough to ask for help.

To accomplish this type of healing is a deep dive into some feelings that have usually been buried a long time. We must acknowledge those parts of us inside that are hurt. We must heal them through practices we learn along the way. Just listening to podcasts or reading a book will not fix it. You absolutely have to get inside yourself, go through the motions, and do the work of healing. You need to do this work with people who are trained in compassion based therapy and have an understanding of trauma.

You see, healing is not an intellectual exercise, it is a feeling transmutation. It is where we discover what lies at the root of our emotions. We then bring it out and heal it, transforming it into something much more beautiful and beneficial to us. Each time we do this, we will discover new things about our past and present. And we will love ourselves a little more.

It is not easy or quick. Although, sometimes you have certain portions heal very swiftly. It takes a commitment, but is so worth it. You have no need to carry this burden with you. It can be lightened off your shoulders to a point where you can move confidently through your life. As you go along on your healing journey, you will feel differently about yourself. You will begin to foster a deep love for the person you are along with respect for the work you have done to overcome tremendous obstacles that were placed upon your life path. When you develop more self love, you will not have a problem expressing your opinions or preferences. You will make better choices in all ways because you truly value yourself.

When we know we are worthy, lovable and have value, we treat ourselves differently. We eat better, try to curb our addictions, and generally show concern about our own welfare on all levels. This self care stemming from self love creates a good balance in our lives and it allows us to free up space to love others more deeply. And that is when really good things start happening for and around us.

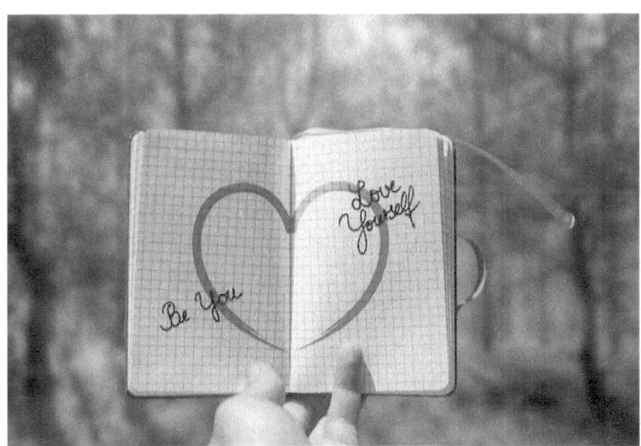

22 - Changing Our World

I am a huge believer that in order to change the world around us, we must first change ourselves. I hold much hope that we can live on a planet where people do not victimize each other. I envision such a world.

Just as a sexual abuse survivor must first come out of their own denial of the events that happened, our population must as well. Often when a person hears about the sexual abuse of another adult, they will raise their voice and sometimes their fist in the air and declare that would never happen to them because ….. of whatever reason they state.

Yet, it does happen each day to people who thought they would react one way and at the time, reacted in another. Unknowingly, when people make these kinds of statements it is condemning to the survivors. It is like saying, if you were like me, you would not have let this happen. Some say of sexual abuse that this would never happen to "their child" as if the children it happened to had poor parenting. The way sexual abuse occurs is complex. It is not black and white but a myriad of shades in between.

The best way to combat this ignorance is to continue telling our stories and having public conversations. We must expose details of how predators work and how they truly prey upon certain situations or people. Revealing their methods is a key prevention tool. Candid conversations with our children are essential. We must let them know they can come and tell us anything. They will not be in trouble, nor will we. We must continually let our children know not to believe anyone that tells them otherwise. Essentially, we must expose the lies.

What do you do when you are no longer a victim and have shed much of your symptoms from the past? Who do you become at this point? Now, you sometimes have anxiety because things are going well and you have to look at rebuilding yourself. This is an interesting angle to think about. Once you get rid of most of your ways that inhibited your life and there are no more toxic people in your circle, you don't want to attract those things into your realm ever again. At this point in your recovery, the truth is you are blooming into your real, precious authentic self and discovering your potential. Look at you — a beautiful work of art.

This is not ….

The End

Go forth and bloom my friend

Visit my website lyraadams.com for

free and paid holistic resources

I would be so grateful if you left a brief written review

wherever you purchased this book!

Appendix

Stages of Healing
Questions from Chapter 4
Please grab a notebook or journal and explore some or all of the following questions. This act will help you clear blockages to your healing.

- Are you hiding your true self in any way?
- Do you lie? Do you go along with others instead of expressing your real feelings because deep down you do not feel your ideas or opinion really count? Are you afraid to speak your mind? Do you lie to yourself?
- Do you have to cover up certain aspects of yourself or can you feel free to live more transparently for all to see?
- Do you fear rejection and does it keep you from having intimate relationships? Have you found yourself ending a relationship before it can get anywhere out of fear of being on the end of rejection later?
- Finish this sentence about your coworkers or friends: If they really knew me,
- Do you feel chronically lonely?
- Do you feel no one really knows you?
- Do you have a parent who shamed you? If so, do they still?
- Have you thought of harming yourself or suicide?
- Do you have self loathing?

Chapter 11 - Preferences
When you are attracting people or situations you do not want, ask questions like:

- What am I feeling inside?
- What mood dominates me now?

- What can I do to set my preferences in this situation?
- What do I fear?
- How can I find balance?

C-PTSD
Eye Movement Desensitization and Reprocessing (EMDR.org)

Addiction Resources
Alcohol - aa.org/
Food - foodaddictsanonymous.org/
Smoking - nicotine-anonymous.org/
Pornography – fightthenewdrug.org

United States Department of Homeland Security Blue Campaign - https://www.dhs.gov/blue-campaign/indicators-human-trafficking.

Report Suspected Human Trafficking - call 1-866-347-2423 Victims may reach out for help by texting HELP or INFO to 233733 (BEFREE) — or they may call 1-888-373-7888.

Recommended Reading
Essential Reiki: A Complete Guide to An Ancient Healing Art by Diane Stein
Wheels of Life by Anodea Judith
Bach Remedies & Flower Essences by Vivien Williamson
Crystal Enlightenment by Katrina Raphaell
Where the Forest Meets the Stars by Glendy Vanderah
When We Believed in Mermaids by Barbara O'Neal

References

Aakvaag, Helene Flood; Thoresen, Siri; Wentzel-Larsen, Tore; Dyb, Grete; Røysamb, Espen; Olff, Miranda. Broken and guilty since it happened: A population study of trauma-related shame and guilt after violence and sexual abuse. *Journal of Affective Disorders*. Volume 204. 2016. Pages 16-23. ISSN 0165-0327. https://doi.org/10.1016/j.jad.2016.06.004.

American Psychiatric Association. (2013). *Diagnostic and statistical manual of mental disorders* (5th ed.). Arlington, VA.

CDC (Centers for Disease Control & Prevention). 2015. Alcohol Poisoning Deaths: A deadly consequence of binge drinking. Retrieved from: https://www.cdc.gov/vitalsigns/alcohol-poisoning-deaths/index.html

Harrison, Patricia Ann, Hoffmann, Norman G. & Edwall, Glenace E. (1989) Differential Drug Use Patterns Among Sexually Abused Adolescent Girls in Treatment for Chemical Dependency, *International Journal of the Addictions*, 24:6, 499-514, DOI: 10.3109/10826088909081832

Liebschutz, Jane et al. 2002. The relationship between sexual and physical abuse and substance abuse consequences. *Journal of Substance Abuse Treatment*, Volume 22, Issue 3, 121 – 128. https://www.journalofsubstanceabusetreatment.com/article/S0740-5472(02)00220-9/fulltext#articleInformation

Marx, Brian P. & Sloan,Denise M. The role of emotion in the psychological functioning of adult survivors of childhood sexual abuse. *Behavior Therapy*, Volume 33, Issue 4, 2002,Pages 563-577. ISSN 0005-7894. https://doi.org/10.1016/S0005-7894(02)80017-X

Monico, Nicolle & Stein, Sophie. June 1, 2020. Effects of Alcohol. https://www.alcohol.org/effects/

New Thinking Allowed With Jeffrey Mishlove. Nov. 14, 2016.The Psychology of Shame with Gerald Loren Fishkin. Video Interview. https://www.youtube.com/watch?v=eH2Qav2rpZ8

Pollock, Anastasia. 2015. The Brain in Defense Mode: How Dissociation Helps Us Survive. https://www.goodtherapy.org/blog/the-brain-in-defense-mode-how-dissociation-helps-us-survive-0429155

Schulze L, Dziobek I, Vater A, et al. Gray matter abnormalities in patients with narcissistic personality disorder. J Psychiatr Res. 2013;47(10):1363-1369. doi:10.1016/j.jpsychires.2013.05.017

Steinberg, Marline & Schnall, Maxine. 2001. *The Stranger In The Mirror*, NY, New York. Harper

Images

Star of Bethlehem Flowers Photo by Eliza28diamonds; Pixabay

Garlic Flowerhead Photo by Alicja; Pixabay

Rose Quartz Photo by WhisperedSecrets; Pixabay

Butterfly on Echinacea – Photo by Deena Creates; Pexels

Aura Image by Doreen Sawitza; Pixabay

Chakra Symbol Illustrations by Peter Lomas; Pixabay

Energy Healing/Reiki Illustration by Mohamed Hassan; Pixabay

Citrine Photograph by Katinkavom Wolfenmond; Pixabay

Singing Bowls Photograph by Magic Bowls; Pixabay

Blue Butterfly Photograph by Garoch; Pixabay

Self Love Journal Photograph by Gerd Altmann; Pixabay

www.ingramcontent.com/pod-product-compliance
Lightning Source LLC
Chambersburg PA
CBHW020902080526
44589CB00011B/410